MEDICAL STATISTICS
from
SCRATCH

MEDICAL STATISTICS
from
SCRATCH

David Bowers
School of Medicine, University of Leeds, UK

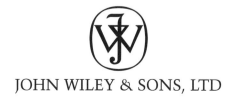

JOHN WILEY & SONS, LTD

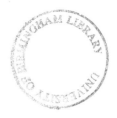

Other Wiley Editorial Offices

John Wiley & Sons, Inc., 111 River Street, Hoboken, NJ 07030, USA

Jossey-Bass, 989 Market Street, San Francisco, CA 94103-1741, USA

Wiley-VCH Verlag GmbH, Boschstr. 12, D-69469 Weinheim, Germany

John Wiley & Sons Australia Ltd, 33 Park Road, Milton, Queensland 4064, Australia

John Wiley & Sons (Asia) Pte Ltd, 2 Clementi Loop #02-01, Jin Xing Distripark,
Singapore 129809

John Wiley & Sons Canada Ltd, 22 Worcester Road, Etobicoke, Ontario, Canada M9W 1L1

Library of Congress Cataloging-in-Publication Data

Bowers, David.
    Medical statistics from scratch / David Bowers.
        p. cm.
    Includes bibliographical references and index.
    ISBN 0-470-84474-4 (alk. paper)
        1. Medical statistics.   2. Medicine—Research—Statistical methods.   I. Title.

    RA409 .B669 2002
    610'.7'27—dc21

                                                            2002029604

British Library Cataloguing in Publication Data

A catalogue record for this book is available from the British Library

ISBN 0-470-84474-4

Typeset in 10/11½ Palatino by Dorwyn Ltd, Rowlands Castle, Hants.
Printed and bound in Great Britain by TJ International, Padstow, Cornwall
This book is printed on acid-free paper responsibly manufactured from sustainable
forestry in which at least two trees are planted for each one used for paper production.

CONTENTS

PREFACE

This book is intended to be an introduction to medical statistics but one which is not too mathematical—in fact has the absolute minimum of maths. The exceptions however are Chapters 17 and 18, on linear and logistic regression. It's really impossible to provide material on these procedures without some maths, and I hesitated about including them at all. However they are such useful and widely used techniques, particularly logistic regression and its production of odds ratios, that I felt they must go in. Of course you don't *have* to read them. It should appeal to anyone training or working in the healthcare arena—whatever their particular discipline—who wants a simple, not-too-technical introduction to the subject. I have aimed the book at:

- students doing either a first degree or diploma in healthcare-related courses
- students doing postgraduate healthcare studies
- healthcare professionals doing professional and membership examinations
- healthcare professionals who want to brush up on some medical statistics generally, or who want a simple reminder of one particular topic
- anybody else who wants to know a bit of what medical statistics is about.

I intended originally to make this book an amalgam of two previous books of mine, *Statistics from Scratch for Health Care Professionals* and *Statistics Further from Scratch*. However, although it covers a lot of the same material as in those two books, this is in reality a completely new book, with a lot of extra stuff, particularly on linear and logistic regression. I am happy to get any comments and criticisms from you. You can e-mail me at: slothist@hotmail.com.

Solutions to the exercises can be obtained from www.wileyeurope.com/go/medical statistics

INTRODUCTION

Before personal computers, researchers had to do most things by hand (by which I mean with a calculator), and so most statistics books were full of equations and their derivations, with many pages of the necessary statistical tables. Analysing anything other than small samples could be time-consuming and error-prone. You also needed to be reasonably good at maths. Of course, for the statistics specialist there is still a need for books which deal with statistical theory, and the often complex mathematics which underlies the subject; but now that computers and their statistics programs are available in most offices and homes, there is room for books which can focus more on an understanding of the principal ideas which underlie the statistical procedures, on knowing which approach is the most appropriate, and under what circumstances, and on the ability to choose a suitable computer program, and then make sense of the results.

So I have tried to keep the technical stuff to a minimum. There are a few equations here and there (mostly in the last couple of chapters), but those I have provided are mainly for the purposes of doing some of the exercises. I have also assumed that readers will have some knowledge of SPSS or Minitab (or some other computer program such as Stata, EpiInfo or BMDP, for example). Short courses in these programs are now widely available to most clinical staff. I also provide a few examples of outputs from SPSS and Minitab, for the commonest applications, which I hope will help you make sense of any results you get. Both SPSS and Minitab have excellent Help facilities which should answer most of the difficulties you may have in the computational process.

Remember this is an introductory book. If you want to explore in more detail any of the methods I describe, you can always turn to one of the comprehensive medical statistics books, such as Altman (1991) or Bland (1995).

I

SOME FUNDAMENTAL STUFF

1

FIRST THINGS FIRST: THE NATURE OF DATA

> **Learning objectives**
>
> When you have finished this chapter you should be able to:
>
> - Explain the difference between nominal, ordinal, and metric discrete and metric continuous variables
> - Identify the type of a variable
> - Explain the non-numeric nature of ordinal data
> - Rank data, and assign values to tied ranks

What is medical statistics?

Medical statistics is a name given to a collection of statistical procedures particularly well-suited to the analysis of healthcare-related data. If you want to answer any but the most trivial questions you will almost certainly need to make use of one or more of them. I am going to examine the most widely used procedures in this book. However, before I can do this, I need to deal first with some basic ideas which relate to the nature of variables and their data and how variables can be classified into a number of distinct types. This material is crucially important in most of what is to follow.

VARIABLES AND DATA

A *variable* is a label we give to something whose value can literally *vary*. For example, *age* is a variable—its value can vary, from individual to individual, or over time. *Sex* is a variable, and can change its value from one person to another.

If you want to know the value or quality of any particular variable, you *observe* it. By "observe", I mean measure it, or count it, or assess it in some way. The value you get from such observing—for example, *age = 48 years*, or *sex = female*—constitutes *data*. Variables (and hence their data) come in three different flavours, which I will discuss in turn.

THE GOOD, THE BAD, AND THE UGLY: TYPES OF VARIABLE

Nominal Categorical Variables

Each data value or quality from a nominal variable can be allocated into one (and only one) of a number of categories. Crucially, these categories *cannot* be put into any meaningful order. For example, *blood type* is a nominal variable, and a value can be allocated to one of four categories:[1] O, A, B, A/B; or B/A, O, A/B; or B, O, A/B, A, or in any other of the possible *arbitrary* ways of arranging four items. Sex is also nominal, with two categories, Male and Female, again with no meaningful order.

Ordinal Categorical Variables

The data from an ordinal variable can also be allocated to one of a number of categories, but crucially the categories *can* now be put in some meaningful order. For example, the variable "Patient satisfaction with nursing care" might have five categories, which could be meaningfully ordered as: "Very unsatisfied", "Unsatisfied", "Neutral", "Satisfied", and "Very satisfied" (or of course in the reverse order—but there *is* an order). Typically, with ordinal variables you will usually have to rely on the judgements or assessments of clinicians, or on the response of patients to questions.

To do any sort of analysis with the patient satisfaction example above (except the most trivial), you will probably need to number the satisfaction categories, for example, as 1, 2, 3, 4, 5, or maybe as –2, –1, 0, 1, 2, or if you think that extreme opinions count for more, as –3, –1, 0, 1, 3. In fact you can use *any* plausible "numbering" sequence, since you don't really know what the actual levels of satisfaction are. In other words, you can't *quantify* these responses accurately, and just because the categories have been numbered doesn't mean that these "numbers" are *real* numbers. How can they be when they can be so arbitrarily defined? To paraphrase Spock, "They're numbers, Jim, but not as we know them."

One crucial consequence is that the difference between one ordinal category and the next is *not necessarily the same*. For example, the difference between the responses "very unsatisfied" and "unsatisfied", and "unsatisfied" and "satisfied", is not necessarily the same. Ordinal values are like the rungs of a ladder whose rungs are not all the same distance apart. Anyone standing on say the fourth rung is certainly higher than someone on the third rung, who in turn is higher than someone on the second rung, but the actual difference in heights between rungs 2 and 3, and between 3 and 4, are not necessarily the same. Nor is someone on rung 4 necessarily twice as high off the ground as someone on rung 2.

All of this means that it is not appropriate to apply any of the rules of basic arithmetic to this sort of data. So, for example, it wouldn't make any sense to calculate the average satisfaction score of 10 patients (by adding the 10 scores together and then dividing by 10, because this involves using addition and division).

---

[1] Four to keep it simple.

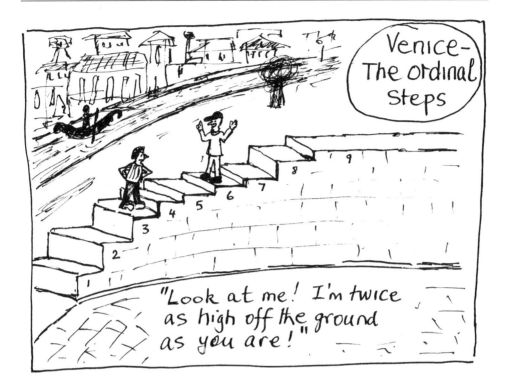

In healthcare research, ordinal data is most often generated by the huge number of clinical *scales* used. To name a few: the Apgar scale (the well-being of neonates), the Beck Depression Inventory scale, the Waterlow Pressure Sore scale, the Glasgow Coma scale (severity of head injury), the Bartel Activities of Daily Living scale (functioning and mobility), and many, many, more! If you are using data from one of these scales, remember that it will be ordinal. Finally, note:

> **MEMO**
>
> Nominal and ordinal variables are known collectively as *categorical variables*.

Metric Variables

With *metric variables* proper measurement is possible. If you have a set of scales you can measure quite accurately the weight (in grams) of a newborn baby, the precision of your measurement depending only on the limitations of the scales. If you have a tape measure you can measure its head circumference (mm), with a clock you can measure its heart rate (in bpm), and you can count quite precisely the number of fingers and toes. In these circumstances a birthweight of 4030g *is* exactly twice as large as a birthweight of 2015g, and the difference between heart rates of 60bpm and 61bpm *is* exactly the same as the difference between values of 61bpm and 62bpm, and so on. Metric data is *truly* numeric—that is, the values can be placed exactly on a proper numeric scale—and because these are real numbers you can apply all of the usual mathematical operations to them. This opens up a much wider range of analytic possibilities than is possible with either nominal or ordinal data.

Ranked Data

Sometimes you may need to *rank* ordinal and numeric data (obviously you can't rank nominal data because its order is completely arbitrary) . This means assigning the largest value a rank of 1 (1st), the next largest a rank of 2 (2nd), and so on. Values that tie are each assigned the average of the ranks they encompass. For example, if you had the nine values 2, 3, 3, 3, 3, 5, 7, 9, 15, you would rank them as: 1, 3.5=, 3.5=, 3.5=, 5, 6, 7, 8, 9, because the four 3s encompass ranks 2, 3, 4 and 5, whose average rank is $(2 + 3 + 4 + 5)/4 = 3.5$. If metric data is ranked, the ranked data becomes *ordinal*—you know that a rank of 1 is higher than a rank of 2, but not by exactly how much.

An example from practice

In a study on priority setting in health authorities, 335 members of the public and 66 general practitioners were asked by a group of district health authorities which of 16 services should be given priority in the budget. The members of the public ranked the following as their top five priorities; the ranks given by the GPs are shown in brackets, who as a matter of interest put community services and care at home (i.e. district nurses) in first place:

1st (5th)	Treatment for children with life-threatening illness (leukaemia)
2nd (4th)	Special care and pain relief for people who are dying (hospices)
3rd (11th)	Medical research for new treatments
4th (12th)	High-technology surgery and procedures for life-threatening conditions (heart or liver transplants)
5th (6th)	Preventative services (screening, immunisation).

Exercise 1.1
Table 1.1 is from a study of GPs' referral rates to hospitals, by speciality and broad age group, in Britain in 1986. Rank the five highest referral rates for the two age groups, 0–14, and 65 and over (1st = highest score). Suggest reasons for any differences in the ranking between the two groups.

WHICH IS WHICH? HOW CAN I TELL?

The easiest way to tell whether data is metric is to check whether its has *units* attached to it, such as: g, kg, mm, m, °C, μ/cm^3, mmHg, seconds, minutes, years, mL, *number of* pressure sores, *number of* deaths, *number of* children, and so on. Notice one important thing about these units—the last three are the result of *counting*: the units are "numbers of things", whereas all the previous units come from *measuring*, where the units differ for each variable. These two different ways

Table 1.1: Referral rates (per 1000 registered patients) to hospitals by speciality and broad age group, in Britain in 1986

	ALL AGES	0–14	15–64	65+
Orthopaedics	8.81	7.25 4	7.88	15.00 4
Psychiatry	5.35	1.50	5.89	8.47
Dermatology	7.85	5.63 6	8.27	9.20
ENT	8.34	12.03 1)	6.29	11.88 5
Medicine	19.27	11.25 ~2	14.94	48.91 1
Rheumatology	8.43	2.18	9.98	10.64 6
Neurology	4.48	3.42	3.93	8.34 7
Gynaecology	9.48	0.43	13.97	3.04
Obstetrics	8.84	0.03	13.83	0.00
Surgery	15.26	8.21 ~3	14.92	26.70 2
Ophthalmology	6.42	5.74 5	4.54	15.41 3
GU	0.52	0.06	0.76	0.13
Urology	4.21	5.07 7	3.07	7.86
All specialities	117.54	74.3	119.6	175.62

of determining the value of a metric variable give rise to two quite distinct types of metric data, *continuous* metric data and *discrete* metric data.

By the way, just because data for a variable is given in integer form (whole numbers) doesn't make it discrete. Continuous metric values are often rounded to the nearest integer for convenience, if there is nothing to be gained from a more precise value. The variable *age* (in years) is nearly always treated this way.

On the other hand, discrete metric data, the result of counting, always comes in integer form. So a woman can have given birth previously to 0 children, or 1 child, or 2 children, etc. but not 1.6 children, or 2.85 children; and similarly, there can be 0 deaths, 1 death, 2 deaths, etc. but not 1.73 deaths. I have summarised the relationship between data types schematically in Figure 1.1.

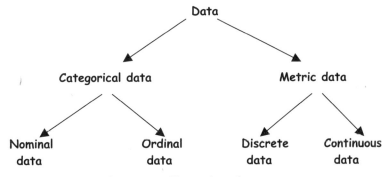

Figure 1.1: The various data types

I would like to emphasise again how important it is to identify the type of data you have before you proceed to any form of analysis. As I said at the beginning of this chapter, choosing a statistical procedure inappropriate to the type of data involved may result in imprecise or, at worst, incorrect results.

Exercise 1.2
List five variables of each type.

[handwritten marginal notes: "nomu al 'Car va / ordual cc I ver / metric vcc / meh cuch / meh desc"]

Exercise 1.3
Table 1.2 contains the characteristics of cases and controls from a case–control study[2] into stressful life events and breast cancer in women. Identify the type of each variable in the table.

Table 1.2: Characteristics of cases and controls from a case–control study into stressful life events and breast cancer in women. Values are mean (SD) unless stated otherwise

VARIABLE	BREAST CANCER GROUP (n = 106)	CONTROL GROUP (n = 226)	p-VALUE
Age *[handwritten: more retad conhnu]*	61.6 (10.9)	51.0 (8.5)	0.000*
Social class† (%): *[handwritten: ordinal]*			
I	10 (10)	20 (9)	
II	38 (36)	82 (36)	
III non-manual	28 (26)	72 (32)	
III manual	13 (12)	24 (11)	0.094‡
IV	11 (10)	21 (9)	
V	3 (3)	2 (1)	
VI	3 (3)	4 (2)	
No. of children (%):			
0	15 (14)	31 (14)	
1	16 (15)	31 (13.7)	0.97
2	42 (40)	84 (37)	
≥3	32 (31)†	80 (35)	
Age at birth of first child	21.3 (5.6)	20.5 (4.3)	0.500*
Age at menarche	12.8 (1.4)	13.0 (1.6)	0.200*
Menopausal state (%):			
Premenopausal	14 (13)	66 (29)	
Perimenopausal	9 (9)	43 (19)	0.000§
Postmenopausal	83 (78)	117 (52)	
Age at menopause	47.7 (4.5)	45.6 (5.2)	0.001*
Lifetime use of oral contraceptives (%)	38	61	0.000‡
No. of years taking oral contraceptive	3.0 (5.4)	4.2 (5.0)	0.065§
No. of months breastfeeding	(n = 90)	(n = 195)	
	7.4 (9.9)	7.4 (12.1)	0.990*
Lifetime use of hormone replacement therapy (%)	29 (27)	78 (35)	0.193§
Mean years of hormone replacement therapy	1.6 (3.7)	1.9 (4.0)	0.460*
Family history of ovarian cancer (%)	8 (8)	10 (4)	0.241§
History of benign breast cancer (%)	15 (15)	105 (47)	0.000§
Family history of breast cancer (%)	16 (15)	35 (16)	0.997§
Units of alcohol/week (%):			
0	38 (36)	59 (26)	
0–4	26 (25)	71 (31)	
5–9	20 (19)	52 (23)	0.927‡
≥ 10	22 (21)	44 (20)	
No. of cigarettes/day			
0	83 (78.3)	170 75.2)	
1–9	8 (7.6)	14 (6.2)	0.383‡
≥ 10	15 (14.2)	42 (18.5)	
Body mass index (kg/m²)	26.8 (5.5)	24.8 (4.2)	0.001*

*Two sample t-test.
†Data for one case missing.
‡χ^2 test for trend.
§χ^2 test.
¶No data for one control.

[2] Don't worry about the different types of study. I discuss them in detail in Chapter 6.

Exercise 1.4

Table 1.3 is from a cross-sectional study to determine the incidence of pregnancy-related venous thromboembolic events and their relationship to selected risk factors, such as maternal age, parity, smoking, and so on. Identify the type of each variable in the table.

Table 1.3: Patient characteristics from a cross-sectional study of thrombotic risk during pregnancy

	THROMBOSIS CASES (n = 608)	CONTROLS (n = 114,940)	OR	95% CI
Maternal age (y) (classification 1)				
≤ 19	26 (4.3)	2817 (2.5)	1.9	1.3, 2.9
20—24	125 (20.6)	23,006 (20.0)	1.1	0.9, 1.4
25–29	216 (35.5)	44,763 (38.9)	1.0	Reference
30–34	151 (24.8)	30,135 (26.2)	1.0	0.8, 1.3
≥ 35	90 (14.8)	14,219 (12.4)	1.3	1.0, 1.7
Maternal age (y) (classification 2)				
≤ 19	26 (4.3)	2817 (2.5)	1.8	1.2, 2.7
20–34	492 (80.9)	97,904 (85.2)	1.0	Reference
≥ 35	90 (14.8)	14,219 (12.4)	1.3	1.0, 1.6
Parity				
Para 0	304 (50.0)	47,425 (41.3)	1.8	1.5, 2.2
Para 1	142 (23.4)	40,734 (35.4)	1.0	Reference
Para 2	93 (15.3)	18,113 (15.8)	1.5	1.1, 1.9
≥ Para 3	69 (11.3)	8429 (7.3)	2.4	1.8, 3.1
Missing data	0 (0)	239 (0.2)		
No. of cigarettes daily				
0	423 (69.6)	87,408 (76.0)	1.0	Reference
1–9	80 (13.2)	14,295 (12.4)	1.2	0.9, 1.5
≥ 10	57 (9.4)	8177 (7.1)	1.4	1.1, 1.9
Missing data	48 (7.9)	5060 (4.4)		
Multiple pregnancy				
No	593 (97.5)	113,330 (98.6)	1.0	Reference
Yes	15 (2.5)	1610 (1.4)	1.8	1.1, 3.0
Preeclampsia				
No	562 (92.4)	111,788 (97.3)	1.0	Reference
Yes	46 (7.6)	3152 (2.7)	2.9	2.1, 3.9
Cesarean delivery				
No	420 (69.1)	102,181 (88.9)	1.0	Reference
Yes	188 (30.9)	12.759 (11.1)	3.6	3.0, 4.3

OR = odds ratio; CI = confidence interval.
Data presented as n (%).

Exercise 1.5

Table 1.4 is from a study to compare two lotions, Malathion and d-phenothrin, in the treatment of head lice, in 193 schoolchildren: 95 children were given Malathion and 98 were given d-phenothrin. Identify the type of each variable in the table.

Table 1.4: Basic characteristics of two groups of children in a study to compare two lotions in the treatment of head lice. One group (95 children) were given Malathion lotion; the second group (98 children) were given d-phenothrin

CHARACTERISTIC	MALATHION (n = 95)	d-PHENOTHRIN (n = 98)
Age at randomisation (yr)	8.6 (1.6)	8.9 (1.6)
Sex—no. of children (%)		
Male	31 (33)	41 (42)
Female	64 (67)	57 (58)
Home		
Number of rooms (mean)	3.3 (1.2)	3.3 (1.8)
Length of hair—no. of children (%)*		
Long	37 (39)	20 (21)
Mid-long	23 (24)	33 (34)
Short	35 (37)	44 (45)
Colour of hair—no. of children (%)		
Blond	15 (16)	18 (18)
Brown	49 (52)	55 (56)
Red	4 (4)	4 (4)
Dark	27 (28)	21 (22)
Texture of hair—no. of children (%)		
Straight	67 (71)	69 (70)
Curly	19 (20)	25 (26)
Frizzy/kinky	9 (9)	4 (4)
Pruritus—no. of children (%)	54 (57)	65 (66)
Excoriations—no. of children (%)	25 (26)	39 (40)
Evaluation of infestation		
Live lice—no. of children (%)		
0	18 (19)	24 (24)
+	45 (47)	35 (36)
++	9 (9)	15 (15)
+++	12 (13)	15 (15)
++++	11 (12)	9 (9)
Viable nits—no. of children (%)*		
0	19 (20)	8 (8)
+	32 (34)	41 (45)
++	22 (23)	24 (25)
+++	18 (19)	20 (21)
++++	4 (4)	4 (4)

The two groups were similar at baseline except for a significant difference for the length of hair (p = 0.02; chi-squared). *One value missing in the d-phenothrin group.

Exercise 1.6

Four migraine patients are asked to assess the severity of their migraine pain one hour after the first symptoms of an attack, by marking a horizontal line, 100mm long. The line is marked "No pain" at the left-hand end, and "Worst possible pain" at the right-hand end. The distance of a patient's mark from the left-hand end is subsequently measured with a rule. Their scores are 25mm, 44mm, 68mm and 85mm. What sort of data is this? Can you calculate the average pain of these four patients? Note that this form of measurement (using a line and getting subjects to mark it) is known as a visual analogue scale (VAS).

At the end of each chapter you should look again at the chapter objectives and satisfy yourself that you have achieved them. continuous?

II

DESCRIBING DATA

2

DESCRIBING DATA WITH TABLES

Learning objectives

When you have finished this chapter you should be able to:

- *Explain what a frequency distribution is*
- *Construct a frequency table from raw data*
- *Construct % frequency, cumulative frequency, and % cumulative frequency tables*
- *Construct grouped frequency tables*
- *Be able to explain what each of the above tables can best be used for*
- *Construct a contingency table, and distinguish it from other similar tables*

FREQUENCY TABLES AND FREQUENCY DISTRIBUTIONS

In Chapter 1 you saw that data comes in two broad types, categorical (nominal and ordinal), and metric (discrete and continuous). In this chapter I want to look at some ways in which data, once you've got it, can be *described*. By "described", I mean identifying the principal features of the data, giving some sort of overall view of its main characteristics, summarising important details, and such like. One way of doing this is to use *tables* and that's what we'll be looking at in this chapter.

When data is first collected it is, like untreated sewage, in its "raw" form. The first thing you want is to get a quick impression of what's going on—the edited high-lights. One possible approach is to organise it in some meaningful way and then put it into a table. For example, suppose you are involved with a study into some aspects of the well-being of newborn infants, and have collected data on five variables for 30 babies chosen at random from those born in a local maternity unit. As a starting point you might begin with a table like that in Table 2.1, which contains all of your raw data but doesn't offer too many insights into what's going on.

For the moment, let's focus on one variable, the Apgar Scale score. This scale, used to assess the well-being of newborn infants, is the sum of the scores on the following five factors:

Heart rate:[1]   Absent = 0; slow (<100) = 1; >100 = 2
Respiratory effort: Absent = 0; weak cry = 1; strong cry = 2

---

[1] This not measured with a stopwatch, but judged from holding the pulse.

Muscle tone: Limp = 0; some flexion = 1; well flexed = 2
Reflex irritability: No response = 0; some motion = 1; cry = 2
Colour   Blue, pale = 0; body pink, extremities blue = 1; all pink = 2

Table 2.1: Raw data on six variables for a sample of 30 infants born in a maternity unit

INFANT NUMBER	BIRTHWEIGHT (g)	APGAR SCORE	SEX	MOTHER SMOKED?	MOTHER'S PARITY
1	3710	8	M	no	1
2	3650	7	F	no	1
3	4490	8	M	no	0
4	3421	6	F	yes	1
5	3399	6	F	no	2
6	4094	9	M	no	3
7	4006	8	M	no	0
8	3287	5	F	yes	5
9	3594	7	F	no	2
10	4206	9	M	no	4
11	3508	7	F	no	0
12	4010	8	M	no	2
13	3896	8	M	no	0
14	3800	8	F	no	0
15	2860	4	M	no	6
16	3798	8	F	no	2
17	3666	7	F	no	0
18	4200	9	M	yes	2
19	3615	7	M	no	1
20	3193	4	F	yes	1
21	2994	5	F	yes	1
22	3266	5	M	yes	1
23	3400	6	F	no	0
24	4090	8	M	no	3
25	3303	6	F	yes	0
26	3447	6	M	yes	1
27	3388	6	F	yes	1
28	3613	7	M	no	1
29	3541	7	M	no	1
30	3886	8	M	yes	1

Best of all would be to put the scores in Table 2.1 into a chart like that in Figure 2.1.

APGAR SCORE	TALLY	NUMBER OF INFANTS (frequency)
4	//	2
5	///	3
6	//// /	6
7	//// //	7
8	//// ///	9
9	///	3

Figure 2.1: Frequency table showing the frequency distribution of Apgar scores for 30 infants born in a maternity unit

Figure 2.1 is called a *frequency table*. The first column contains the variable's possible categories or values. The second column, labelled "Tally", is the column I used to help me record which category each value went in as I worked through the raw data, and doesn't appear in the final table. The third column, labelled "frequency", records the number of subjects or items in each category. A frequency table gives us a picture of the *frequency distribution* of a variable. With Figure 2.1 you get a much clearer view of the main features of the data than with Table 2.1. You can see immediately that: a lot of the infants had Apgar scores towards the top of the range, with fewer values below 7; the commonest score is 8 (nine infants); and the largest score is 9—but with only three infants. In this sense you have *described* some interesting characteristics of the data.

An Example from Practice

We can construct frequency tables for any type of variable. For example, Table 2.2 shows the frequency distribution for the variable *level of satisfaction* with their psychiatric nursing by 475 psychiatric in-patients. The variable has five categories as shown. The frequency values in the middle column indicate that most of the patients were happy with their psychiatric nurses. In total 282 patients (121 + 161), out of 475, more than half, were either very satisfied or satisfied. Much smaller numbers expressed dissatisfaction.

Table 2.2: The frequency and relative freqency distributions for the variable "level of satisfaction" with nursing care by 475 psychiatric in-patients

SATISFACTION WITH NURSING CARE	NO. OF PATIENTS	PERCENTAGE
Very satisfied	121	25.5
Satisfied	161	33.9
Neutral	90	18.9
Dissatisfied	51	10.7
Very dissatisfied	52	10.9

Relative Frequency

Helpfully, Table 2.2 also contains a third column of *% frequencies* (also known as *relative* frequencies). These show, not the number of patients in each category, but their percentage of the total. Thus you can see that 25.5% were very satisfied and 33.9% satisfied. Only 10.9% were very unsatisfied. Working these percentages out for yourself would have been a pain—relative frequencies are helpful to readers, who will usually be more interested in broad patterns rather than with the actual numbers. If possible, always provide them.

Exercise 2.1
The data below are the *parity* (the number of previous live births) of 40 women chosen at random from the 332 women in the stress and breast cancer study referred to in Exercise

1.4. (a) Construct frequency and relative frequency tables. (b) Describe briefly what is revealed about the principal features of parity in these women.

    4 0 2 3 2 2 3 3 0 3 1 2 8 3 4 2 1 2 2 2
    2 2 3 2 2 3 0 3 2 4 0 1 3 5 1 1 0 3 2 1

Cumulative Frequency

Suppose you now wanted to know the number, or percentage, of infants who had an Apgar score of *less* than 7, i.e. of 6 or less. A comparatively quick way of getting this information is to add up, or *cumulate*, the frequency (or % frequency) Apgar values, starting at the top of the table and working down. Doing this with the data in Figure 2.1 gives the cumulative frequency and relative cumulative frequency values shown in the last two columns of Table 2.3.

Table 2.3: Cumulative and percentage cumulative frequencies for the Apgar scores from the raw data in Table 2.1

APGAR SCORE	NUMBER OF INFANTS (frequency)	PERCENTAGE OF INFANTS (relative frequency)	CUMULATIVE NUMBER OF INFANTS (cumulative frequency)	CUMULATIVE PERCENTAGE OF INFANTS (relative cumulative frequency)
4	2	6.67	2	6.67
5	3	10.00	5	16.67
6	6	20.00	11	36.67
7	7	23.33	18	60.00
8	9	30.00	27	90.00
9	3	10.00	30	100.00

The cumulative frequency for each category tells us how many (or what percentage of) subjects there are in that category *and in all the categories above it*, i.e. with a smaller value, in the table. For example, the last two columns tell us that six infants had a score of 6, and 36.67% had a score of 6 or less, i.e. below 7. A cumulative frequency table provides us with a different view of the data. Moreover it allows us to draw a useful chart, as you will see in Chapter 3. Note that although you can legitimately calculate cumulative frequencies for both metric and ordinal data, it makes no sense to do so for nominal data, because of the arbitrary category order.

Exercise 2.2
(a) Add cumulative and relative cumulative frequency columns to the frequency table you constructed in Exercise 2.1 for the parity data. (b) What percentage of women had a parity score of (i) 2, (ii) greater than 2?

Grouped Frequency

Frequency tables work best for ordinal and discrete metric data. With continuous metric data there are often too many values to make these tables of any practical

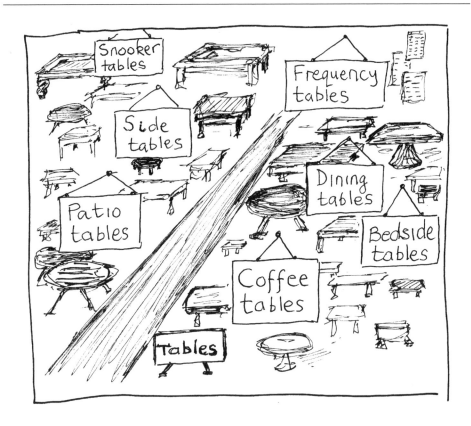

use. As an illustration, consider the birthweight data in Table 2.1. Birthweight (g) is a metric continuous variable, although it has been recorded here in integer form, greater precision not being necessary. Among the 30 infants there are *none* with the same birthweight, and a frequency table with 30 rows and a frequency of 1 in every row would add very little to what you already know from the raw data (apart from telling you what the minimum and maximum birthweights are). One solution is to *group* the data into, if possible, *equal*-sized groups, to produce a *grouped frequency distribution*.

Choosing the number and width of the groups is a matter of trial and error. You want enough groups to be helpful, but not so many that you end up with only a few values in each group. On the other hand, too few groups will conceal too much detail. As a rule of thumb, "no fewer than four or five groups, no more than eight or nine" seems about right. You also need enough data values to make the exercise worthwhile; the 30 here are barely enough, but in real life there will hopefully be more.

A helpful approach is to first determine the difference between the largest and smallest value (this is known as the *range*). For example, with the birthweight data, the range is 4490g minus 2860g = 1630g. With say five groups we get a group width of 1630/5 = 326g, so we could make each group 300g wide (I would have preferred a group width of 500g, but this doesn't give me enough groups). By the way, if your data has decimal places, your group limits will need to reflect this.

This gives groups (or classes) of 2700–2999, 3000–3299, etc. Groups are more properly referred to as *classes*, and the bottom value of each class or group is known as the *class lower limit*, the top value the *class upper limit*. So 2700g is the *class lower limit* of the first class, and 2999g the *class upper limit*. It's then just a matter of counting how many of the data values fall in each group and entering these values in the second column (or getting a computer program to do it). If possible, keep all of your group widths the same, but if you find that a lot of the values fall into just one or two groups you might need to try different group widths; e.g. divide some groups into two.

The resulting grouped frequency table for birthweight is shown in Table 2.4. This provides a better description of the data's main features than did the raw data. For example, you can now see that most of the infants had a birthweight around the middle of the range of values, with fewer at either end. You can still calculate cumulative and relative cumulative from grouped frequencies if you wish.

Table 2.4: Grouped freqency distribution for birthweight (g) of 30 infants (data in Table 2.1)

BIRTHWEIGHT (g)	NO. OF INFANTS (frequency)
2700–2999	2
3000–3299	3
3300–3599	9
3600–3899	9
3900–4199	4
4200–4499	3

Open-ended Groups

One problem arises when one or two values are a long way from the general mass of the data, either much lower or much higher. These values are called *outliers*, and their presence can mean having lots of empty or near-empty frequency cells at one or both ends of the table. For example, one infant with a birthweight of 6050g would mean having five empty cells before this value is recorded. One favoured solution is to use *open-ended* groups. If you define a new last group as ≥5000g, you can record a frequency of 1 in this frequency cell,[2] and thus incorporate all of the intervening empty groups into this single one.

Both of the two grouped age distributions in Table 1.3 use open-ended classes at both ends of the distribution, ≤19 and ≥35. One problem is that if you don't have access to the raw data you may have little idea what any of the values in these open-ended groups actually are, although usually you can place some sort of practical limits on them. For example, this is a study of *maternal* events, so you know that the earliest possible age is around 12–ish, and the oldest age possibly 50.

Exercise 2.3
The data in Table 2.5 is from a cohort study to ascertain the extent of variation in the case-mix of adult admissions to intensive care units (ICUs) in Britain and Ireland, and its impact on outcomes. The table records the percentage mortality in 26 intensive care units. Construct a grouped frequency table of percentage mortality.

---

[2] ≥ means greater than or equal to; ≤ means less than or equal to.

Table 2.5: Percentage mortality in 26 intensive care units from a cohort study to describe the extent of variation in the case-mix of adult admissions to such units in Britain and Ireland, and its impact on outcomes

ICU	1	2	3	4	5	6	7	8	9	10	11	12	13
MORTALITY %	15.2	31.3	14.9	16.3	19.3	18.2	20.2	12.8	14.7	29.4	21.1	20.4	13.6

ICU	14	15	16	17	18	19	20	21	22	23	24	25	26
MORTALITY %	22.4	14.0	14.3	22.8	26.7	18.9	13.7	17.7	27.2	19.3	16.1	13.5	11.2

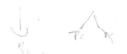

CROSS-TABULATION

The frequency tables above provide us with a description of the frequency distribution of *single* variables. Sometimes, however, you will want to examine the association between *two* variables, within a *single* group of individuals. You can do this by presenting the data in a table of *cross-tabulation*, in which the rows represent the categories of one variable, and the columns represent the categories of a second variable. These tables can provide some insights into *sub-group* structures. By a "sub-group" I mean smaller identifiable groups within the overall group, such as male infants and female infants among all infants.

To illustrate the idea, let's return to the 30 infants whose data is recorded in Table 2.1. Suppose you are particularly interested in a possible association between infants with Apgar score of less than 7 (since this is an indicator for potential problems in the infant's well-being), and whether the mother smoked or not (yes or no). Notice that we have only one group here, the 30 infants, but two sub-groups, infants with Apgar scores of less than 7 and those with a score of 7 or more. With two nominal variables, each with two categories, you will need a cross-tabulation with two rows, and two columns, giving you four cells. You then need to go through the raw data in Table 2.1 and count the number of infants to be allocated to each cell. The final result is shown in Table 2.6.

Table 2.6: A cross-tabulation of the variables "Mother smoked?" and "Apgar score <7?" for 30 newborn infants

MOTHER SMOKED?	APGAR <7		
	Yes	No	Totals
Yes	8	2	10
No	3	17	20
Totals	11	19	30

Quite obviously, Table 2.6 is much more informative than the raw data. You can see immediately that 10 out of the 30 babies had mothers who smoked, and that 11 out of 30 babies had Apgar scores <7. Moreover, of these 11 babies, the number with mothers who smoked is four times as large as those with non-smoking mothers (8 compared to 2). More helpful would be a cross-tabulation with *percentage* values. Table 2.7 shows the data in Table 2.6 expressed as percentages of the *column* totals, and you can see that 73% of infants with low Apgar scores had mothers who had smoked, compared with only 23% with mothers who hadn't.

These results might provoke you into thinking that maybe there's a link of some sort between these two variables. Note that when appropriate you can also express the cross-tabulation with values as percentages of the *row* totals.

Table 2.7:   A cross-tabulation of the variables "Apgar score <7?" and "Mother smoked during pregnancy?", for 30 newborn infants, with values expressed as percentages of the *column* totals

MOTHER SMOKED?	APGAR <7	
	Yes	*No*
Yes	73	10
No	27	90
Totals	100	100

Tables 2.6 and 2.7 are often called *contingency tables*. A contingency table represents only *one* group of individuals, but separated into *sub-groups*, as with the smoking and with non-smoking mothers.

Exercise 2.4

The diagnosis (breast lump benign = 0; breast lump malignant = 1), for the same 40 women (in the same order) as in Exercise 2.1, is shown below. (a) Cross-tabulate diagnosis against parity (with categories "2 or fewer children" and "more than two children"). (b) Repeat expressing the values as percentages. (c) What does the cross-tabulation reveal, if anything, about an association between diagnosis and parity?

      0 0 0 0 0 1 0 0 0 0 0 1 1 1 0 0 1 0 0 1 . . .
      . . . 0 0 0 0 0 0 0 1 0 0 0 0 0 1 0 0 0 0 0 0

TABLES THAT ARE NOT CONTINGENCY TABLES

Table 2.8 shows the outcome (alive or dead), 12 months after some clinical event, for *two* groups of patients, males and females, recruited separately and without reference to each other by two health visitors. This table is *not* a contingency table, because two quite separate groups of individuals are involved.

Table 2.8:   A table that is *not* a contingency table, because more than one group of individuals are involved, in this case males and females

OUTCOME	GROUP 1 (males)	GROUP 2 (females)
Alive	55	70
Dead	5	10
Totals	60	80

Exercise 2.5

Look back at Table 1.2 from the life stress and breast cancer study. Construct a suitable 2-by-2 table, in percentage terms, with the columns being *Cases* (breast cancer), and *Controls* (no breast cancer), and the rows *Lifetime use of oral contraceptives, OCP* (yes or no). Comment on any patterns you can see in the table. Is this a contingency table?

3

DESCRIBING DATA WITH CHARTS

Learning objectives

When you have finished this chapter you should be able to:

- *Choose the most appropriate chart for a given data type*
- *Draw pie charts, and simple, clustered and stacked bar charts*
- *Draw dotplots and histograms, and explain the area properties of the histogram*
- *Draw step charts and ogives*
- *Draw time-series charts*
- *Interpret and explain what a chart reveals*

Picture It!

In terms of describing data, of seeing "what's going on", an appropriate chart is always a good idea. What "appropriate" means depends primarily on the *type* of data, as well as on what particular features of it you want to explore. In this chapter I am going to examine some of the commonest charts available for describing data, and indicate which charts are appropriate for each type of data in turn. Apart from the dotplot, I produced all of the charts in this chapter using Microsoft Word 2000's own chart function, which is (as far as I know) identical to Excel's chart function.

CHARTING NOMINAL DATA

The Pie Chart

You may know what a *pie chart* is. Each segment (slice) of a pie chart is proportional to the size, the frequency, of the category it represents. For example, Figure 3.1 is a pie chart of hair colour for the children receiving Malathion in the nit lotion study in Table 1.4. I have chosen to display the percentage values, which are often more helpful. If (unlikely) you have to draw a pie chart by hand, the angle subtended at the centre by each category segment is equal to the proportion of the total number of subjects in that category, times $360°$. For example, the angle for blonde children is $(15/95) \times 360 = 57°$.

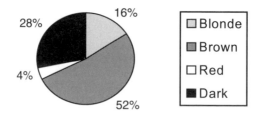

Figure 3.1: Pie chart of hair colour of children receiving Malathion (in Table 3.1)

A few other points about pie charts:

- Don't use them to represent more than four or five categories at the most, otherwise getting a clear picture becomes more difficult.
- Pie charts can represent only one variable (in this example, hair colour). You will therefore need a separate pie chart for each variable you want to chart. Strictly speaking, if you want to compare two or more samples of different size using a number of pie charts, the area of each chart should be proportional to the total frequency (of each sample).
- If practicable, put the segments in the same order as any accompanying table, and start at 0°.

An Example from Practice

The two pie charts in Figure 3.2, taken from a study to investigate the causes of stroke in patients with asymptotic internal carotid artery stenosis, show the percentages of disabling and non-disabling ipsilateral strokes for a number of causes, within the two categories <60% stenosis and 60–90% stenosis. The pie charts are self-explanatory; for example, the largest cause of both disabling and non-disabling stroke was of large-artery origin.

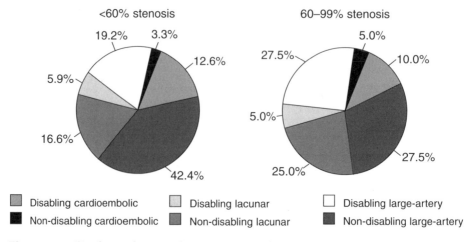

Figure 3.2: Pie charts showing the percentages of disabling and non-disabling ipsilateral strokes for each cause, within the two categories of <60% stenosis and 60–90% stenosis, taken from a cohort study to investigate the causes of stroke in patients with asymptotic internal carotid artery stenosis

The Simple Bar Chart

An alternative to the pie chart for nominal data is the *bar chart*. Figure 3.3 is a *simple* bar chart of hair colour for the group of nit-lotion children, with frequency on the vertical or *y* axis, and the categories on the horizontal or *x* axis. Although frequency is most commonly plotted, other measures can be displayed in this way—for example, rates, ratios, prevalences, and so on. Some points about bar charts:

- The bars should all be the same *width*.
- There should be equal spaces between bars—these emphasise the categorical nature of the data.
- It sometimes helps if the bars are drawn in ascending or descending height (if this is possible).

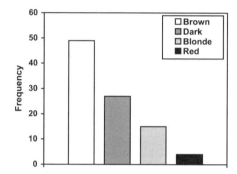

Figure 3.3: Simple bar chart of hair colour of children receiving Malathion in the nit-lotion study

Exercise 3.1
Use the data in Table 1.4 to sketch (a) a pie chart, and (b) a simple bar chart, showing the hair colour of the children receiving *d*-phenothrin.

The Clustered Bar Chart

If you have more than one variable or group you can use the *clustered* bar chart. Suppose you also know the *sex* of the children receiving Malathion in the above example. This gives us two groups, boys and girls, with the data shown in Table 3.1.

Table 3.1: Frequency distribution of hair colour by sex of Malathion children in the nit-lotion study

HAIR COLOUR	FREQUENCY	
	Boys	*Girls*
Blonde	4	11
Brown	29	20
Red	1	3
Dark	14	13

There are two ways of presenting a clustered bar chart. Figure 3.4 shows one configuration, with hair colour categories on the horizontal axis, which is helpful if you want to compare the relative sizes of the groups *within each category* (e.g. red-haired boys versus red-haired girls).

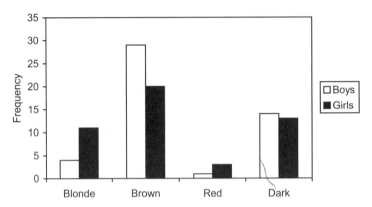

Figure 3.4: Clustered bar chart of hair colour by sex for children in Table 3.1

A different format is shown in Figure 3.5, which would be more useful if you wanted to compare category sizes *within each group*—for example, red-haired girls compared to dark-haired girls. Neither chart is better than the other: it depends on what aspect of the data you want to examine. Clustered bar charts work fine provided you use them only when the number of categories is reasonably small— remember these charts are supposed to be helpful and quickly interpreted.

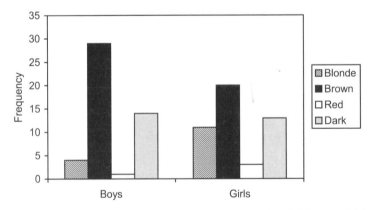

Figure 3.5: Clustered bar chart of sex by hair colour for children in Table 3.1

Exercise 3.2
Use the data in Table 1.4 to sketch a clustered percentage bar chart showing the hair colour of children receiving Malathion and d-phenothrin. There are two possible formats. Explain why you chose the one you did.

An Example from Practice

The clustered bar chart in Figure 3.6 is from a study describing the development and validation of the APACHE II scale, a severity-of-disease classification scale to measure risk of death, and used mainly in ICUs. APACHE II has a range of 0 (least risk of death) to 71 (greatest risk of death). Data was available on 5815 ICU patients, one group admitted to an ICU for medical emergencies, the second admitted directly to ICU following surgery. The bar chart shows the percentage death rate (vertical axis), against bands of the APACHE II score. Quite clearly, for those less severely ill, percentage mortality among the medical emergency group is noticeably higher than among the post-operative group. For those patients classified as the most severely ill (scores of 35+), the situation is reversed.

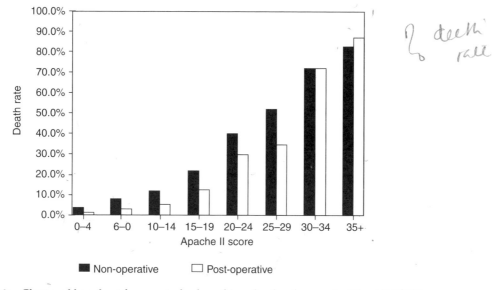

Figure 3.6: Clustered bar chart from a study describing the development of the APACHE II scale, a severity of disease scale for ICUs, with a range of 0 (well) to 71 (dead). Data is available on two groups of patients, one of patients admitted to an ICU for medical emergencies, the second admitted directly to ICU following surgery. The vertical axis is death rate (%)

The Stacked Bar Chart

Figure 3.7 shows a *stacked* bar chart for the same hair colour and sex data shown in Figure 3.5. Instead of appearing side-by-side, the bars are now stacked on top of each other. I could, alternatively, have used four columns for the four colour categories, with two groups per column (boys and girls). Again it depends on what you want to compare. Stacked bar charts are good if you want to compare the *total* number of subjects in each group (total number of boys and girls for example), but not so good if you want to compare category sizes *between* groups (e.g. red-haired girls with red-haired boys).

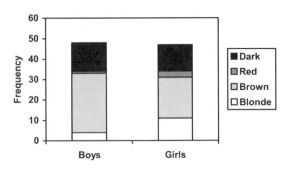

Figure 3.7: A stacked bar chart of hair colour and sex

CHARTING ORDINAL DATA

The Pie Chart

You can also use a pie chart to represent the categories of an ordinal variable, with the same proviso—don't attempt to represent too many categories.

The Bar Chart

Bar charts are used in exactly the same way with ordinal categories as with nominal categories, but ordinal variables will usually have more categories, sometimes too many to create a useful bar chart—in which case, values can be grouped and the groups charted.

Exercise 3.3
Sketch a clustered bar chart for the menopausal status of the women in both groups in Table 1.2. Comment on what is revealed.

Exercise 3.4
The data in Table 3.2 is taken from a cross-section study to investigate duration of breast feeding and arterial distensibility leading to cardiovascular disease. The table describes the basic characteristics of two groups, 149 subjects who were bottle-fed as infants, and 182 who were breast-fed. Sketch a clustered bar chart of the percentage number of subjects in each smoking category for both groups, and comment on what is revealed. Do you think I am justified in treating smoking history as an ordinal variable? Explain.

The Dotplot

In practice, you'll probably use a computer program to draw your charts. Apart from Word and Excel, there are many dedicated statistics programs, such as SPSS and Minitab, which will also do the job as well or better. One very useful chart is the *dotplot*. Unfortunately, only Minitab among the aforementioned programs has the dotplot in its repertoire. Figure 3.8 is a Minitab dotplot of the Apgar scores in Figure 2.1, with a column of dots, equal in number to the frequency, for each Apgar value on the horizontal axis. The dotplot is particularly useful with ordinal variables if the number of categories is too large for a bar chart.

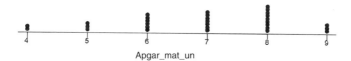

Figure 3.8: Dotplot of the Apgar scores in Figure 2.1

Table 3.2: Data from a cross-section study to investigate duration of breast-feeding and arterial distensibility leading to cardiovascular disease. Values are mean (SD or range) unless stated otherwise

VARIABLE	BREAST-FED	BOTTLE-FED	P-VALUE FOR DIFFERENCE BETWEEN GROUPS
No. of participants (men/women)	149 (67/82)	182 (93/89)	—
Age (years)	23 (20 to 28)	23 (20 to 27)	0.07
Height (cm)	170 (10)	168 (9)	0.03
Weight (kg)	70.4 (14.5)	68.7 (13.1)	0.28
Body mass index (kg/m²)	24.2 (4.1)	24.3 (3.7)	0.83
Length of breast-feeding (months)	3.33 (0 to 18)	—	—
Resting arterial diameter (mm)	3.32 (0.59)	3.28 (0.59)	0.45
Distensibility coefficient (mm Hg^{-1})	0.133 (0.07)	0.140 (0.08)	0.38
Cholesterol (mmol/L)	4.43 (0.99)	4.61 (1.01)	0.11
LDL cholesterol (mmol/L)	2.71 (0.88)	2.90 (0.93)	0.07
HDL cholesterol (mmol/L)	1.18 (0.25)	1.18 (0.31)	0.96
Systolic blood pressure (mmHg)	128 (14)	128 (14)	0.93
Diestolic blood pressure (mmHg)	70 (9)	71 (8)	0.31
Smoking history (%)			
Smokers	49 (33)	64 (35)	
Former smokers	25 (17)	22 (12)	0.78
Non-smokers	75 (50)	96 (53)	
No. (%) in social class:			
I	12 (8)	13 (7)	
II	36 (24)	33 (18)	
IIINM	51 (34)	62 (34)	0.19
IIIM	24 (16)	36 (20)	
IV	22 (15)	33 (18)	
V	4 (3)	5 (3)	

LDL = low density lipoprotein, HDL = high density lipoprotein

CHARTING DISCRETE METRIC DATA

A dotplot works well with discrete metric data. A bar chart can and often is used but remember that the category values—for example, parity scores such as, 0, 1, 2, etc.—are "point" values. It's not possible to have slightly less than 2 children, its either 2 children or 1 child. So instead of using bars (which have a *width*), you should really use vertical *lines*. Unfortunately, most computer programs I am aware of won't give you this sort of chart, so the next best thing is to make your bars as thin as possible!

An Example from Practice

Figure 3.9 is an example of a bar chart used to present *numbers* of measles cases (discrete metric data), in 23 schools in Kentucky in a school year.

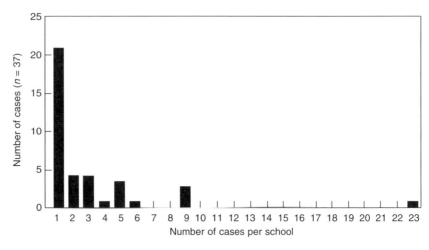

Figure 3.9:   Bar chart used to represent discrete metric data on numbers of measles cases in 23 schools. Sept 1991–July 1992

CHARTING CONTINUOUS METRIC DATA
The Histogram

As you have seen, a continuous metric variable can take a very large number of values, so it is usually impractical to plot them (although it's possible to use a dotplot if the data is recorded in integer form, as age often is for example). Because of this, metric continuous data is often *grouped* before being charted with a *histogram*. A histogram looks like a bar chart but without gaps between adjacent bars. This emphasises the continuous nature of the underlying variable[1]. If possible, try to keep the size or width of each group the same, although this won't always be appropriate if in so doing a large proportion of the values fall into one (or a few) groups, or if you are particularly interested in smaller grouping over selected parts of the data.

One limitation of the histogram is that it can represent only one variable (like the pie chart), and this can make comparisons between two histograms inconvenient. If you try to plot more than one histogram on the same axes, invariably parts of one chart will overlap, or be overlapped, by the other chart.

One important property of the histogram is that its total area (width × height of *all* the bars added together) is proportional to total frequency. If your groups are *not* all of the same width, you need to be cautious. With equal-sized groups, all the widths are the same, so the height of each bar is equal to its group frequency. However, if say one of the groups is *twice as wide* as the other groups, then to preserve the area property, the frequency of this group (i.e. the height of the corresponding bar) has to be *halved*. Conversely, if a group is only *half as wide*, its frequency has to be *doubled*, and so on. You might need to take this into account when you are entering data into a computer program to draw a histogram.

---

[1] To draw a histogram with Word, create a simple bar chart, then use the Column Chart option, select one of the bars, click Format>Format Selected Data Series>Options> set Gap Width = 0.

Dealing with Open-ended Classes

Many published grouped frequency tables have "open-ended" groups or *classes* (as they are formally known), about which some assumption has to be made before the histogram can be drawn. The problem is illustrated in Table 3.3, which shows the body mass index (BMI) of 7270 middle-aged British men in the British Regional Heart Study of cardiovascular disease. The focus of this particular investigation was serum potassium level, smoking and mortality. The authors have used an open-ended class both at the top of the table (BMI <22) and at the bottom (BMI ≥28).

Table 3.3: Body mass index of 7270 middle-aged British men in the British Regional Heart Study

BODY MASS INDEX	NUMBER
<22	948
22–23.9	1466
24–25.9	1973
26–27.9	1528
≥28	1355

Before you can interpret or draw a histogram you have to make some sensible assumption about the width of any open-ended groups. You might decide that a realistic minimum value for body mass index in Table 3.3 is 16, and a maximum 38 (you could always refer to some standard reference values for better information). This means the two open-ended classes could be 16–21 and 28–38.

Exercise 3.5
Sketch separate histograms for the percentage age distribution of pregnant women (classification 1), for both cases and controls, for the data shown in Table 1.3. Justify any assumptions and comment on what the histograms reveal.

Another Example from Practice

The histogram in Figure 3.10 is from the same British Regional Heart Study as Table 3.3 and shows the serum potassium level (mmol/L) of the men not receiving treatment for hypertension.

Exercise 3.6
Comment on what the histogram in Figure 3.10 reveals about serum potassium levels in this sample of 7262 British men.

Exercise 3.7
The grouped age data in Table 3.4 is from a study to identify predictive factors for suicide, and shows the age distribution by sex of 974 subjects who attempted suicide unsuccessfully, and those among them who were later successful. Sketch separate histograms of percentage age for the *male* attempters and later succeeders. Comment on what the charts show.

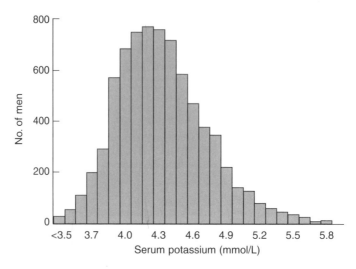

Figure 3.10: Histrogram of the serum potassium levels (mmol/L) of 7662 British men aged 40–59 years, from the British Regional Heart Study, a cohort study of cardiovascular disease

Table 3.4: Grouped age data from a follow-up cohort study to identify predictive factors for suicide

	NO. (%) ATTEMPTING SUICIDE		NO. (%) LATER SUCCESSFUL	
	Men (n = 412)	Women (n = 562)	Men (n = 48)	Women (n = 55)
Age (years)				
15–24	57 (13.8)	80 (14.2)	3 (6.3)	3 (5.5)
25–34	131 (31.8)	132 (23.5)	10 (20.8)	12 (21.8)
35–44	103 (25.0)	146 (26.0)	16 (33.3)	16 (29.1)
45–54	62 (15.0)	90 (16.0)	11 (22.9)	9 (16.4)
55–64	38 (9.2)	58 (10.3)	4 (8.3)	4 (7.3)
65–74	18 (4.4)	43 (7.7)	3 (6.3)	8 (14.5)
75–84	1 (0.2)	11 (2.0)	0	2 (3.6)
>85	2 (0.5)	2 (0.4)	1 (2.1)	1 (1.8)
Living alone	96 (23.3)	85 (15.1)	17 (35.4)	14 (25.5)
Employed	139 (33.7)	185 (32.9)	14 (29.2)	13 (23.6)

CHARTING CUMULATIVE ORDINAL OR DISCRETE METRIC DATA

The Step Chart

You can chart *cumulative* ordinal data or *cumulative* discrete metric data (data for both types of variables is integer) with a *step chart*. In a step chart the total height of each step from the horizontal axis represents the cumulative frequency, up to and including that category or value. The height of each individual step is the frequency of the corresponding category or value.

An Example from Practice

Figure 3.11 is a step chart of the cumulative rate of suicide (number per 1000 of the population), in 152 Swedish municipalities, taken from a study into the use of calcium-channel blockers (prescribed for hypertension) and the risk of suicide. So for example, by year 4 the suicide rate per 1000 of the population was 7 minus 5.2 = 1.8 (the approximate height of the step), and the cumulative suicide rate in the study group had risen to 7 per thousand. You can produce step charts for numeric ordinal data, such as cumulative Apgar scores, in exactly the same way.

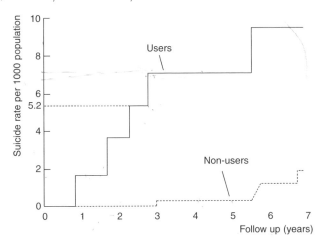

Figure 3.11:   Step chart of the cumulative rate of suicide (number per 1000 of the population) in 152 Swedish municipalities, taken from a study into the use of calcium-channel blockers (prescribed for hypertension) and the risk of suicide

Exercise 3.8
Draw a step chart for the percentage cumulative Apgar scores in Table 2.3.

CHARTING CUMULATIVE METRIC CONTINUOUS DATA
The Cumulative Frequency Curve or Ogive

With continuous metric data, there is assumed to be a smooth *continuum* of values, so you can chart cumulative frequency with a correspondingly smooth curve, known as a *cumulative frequency curve*, or *ogive*. If you add columns for cumulative and relative cumulative frequency to the birthweight data to Table 2.4, you get Table 3.5.

If you want to draw an ogive by hand, you plot, for each group or class, the group cumulative, or percentage cumulative frequency value, against the *lower* limit of the next *higher* group. So, for example, 16.67 is plotted against 3300, 46.67 against 3600, and so on.[2] The points should be joined with a smooth curve. The result is

---

[2] To be technical, each cumulative frequency value should be plotted against the point half-way between the upper class limit of its own group and the lower class limit of the next higher group (this value is known as the "group upper boundary"). So 16.67 would be plotted against 3299.5, the upper boundary of the 3000–3299 group. But our approximation is generally thought close enough—and a lot less complicated!

Table 3.5: Cumulative and relative cumulative freqency for the birthweight data in Table 2.4

BIRTHWEIGHT (g)	NO. OF INFANTS (frequency)	PERCENTAGE CUMULATIVE FREQUENCY
2700–2999	2	6.67
3000–3299	3	16.67
3300–3599	9	46.67
3600–3899	9	76.67
3900–4199	4	90.00
4200–4499	3	100.00

shown in Figure 3.12. Notice that I have put a percentage cumulative frequency of 0 in the imaginary group 2400–2699g. This enables me to close the ogive at the left-hand end.

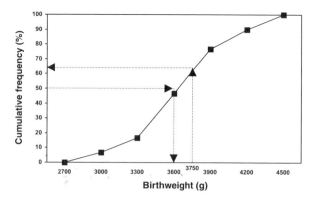

Figure 3.12:   The relative cumulative frequency curve (or ogive) for the percentage cumulative birthweight data in Table 3.5

The ogive can be very useful if you want to estimate the cumulative frequency for any value on the horizontal axis, which is not one of the original class limit values. For example, suppose you want to know what percentage of infants had a birth-weight of 3750g or less. By drawing a line vertically upwards from a value of 3750g on the horizontal axis to the ogive, and then horizontally to the vertical axis, you can estimate a percentage cumulative frequency of about 63%. So about 63% of the infants weighed 3750g or less. You can of course ask such questions in reverse: for example, what birthweight marks the lowest 50% of birthweights? This time you would start with a value of 50% on the vertical axis, move right to the ogive, then down to the value of about 3600g on the horizontal axis.

An Example from Practice

Figure 3.13 shows two percentage cumulative frequency ogives for total cholesterol concentration in two groups, taken from a study into the effectiveness of health checks conducted by nurses in primary care.

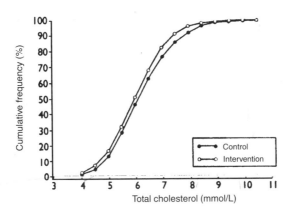

Figure 3.13: Percentage cumulative frequency curves for total cholesterol concentration in two groups

Exercise 3.9

(a) Comment on what Figure 3.13 reveals about the cholesterol levels in the two groups.
(b) Sketch percentage cumulative frequency curves of age for the male suicide attempters and later succeeders, shown in Table 3.1 (see also Exercise 3.7). What age divides each group into equal numbers of subjects?

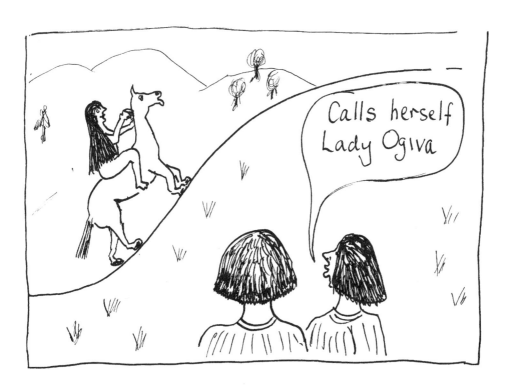

CHARTING TIME-BASED DATA: THE TIME-SERIES CHART

If the data you have collected come from measurements made at regular intervals of time (minutes, weeks, years, etc.), you can describe the changes over time with a *time-series chart*. Usually these charts are used with metric data, but they may also be appropriate for ordinal data. Time is always plotted on the horizontal axis and data values on the vertical axis.

An Example from Practice

Figure 3.14 shows the suicide rates (number of suicides per one million of population), for males and females aged 15–29 years in England and Wales, between 1974 and 1999. The contrasting patterns in the male/female rates are very obvious, and more impactful perhaps than a table of values.

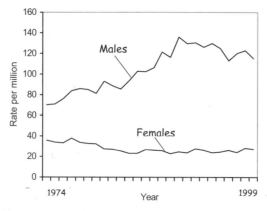

Figure 3.14: Suicide rates (number of suicides per one million of population), for males and females aged 15–29 years in England and Wales, between 1974 and 1999

There is one other useful chart, the *boxplot*, but that will have to wait until I have introduced some new ideas in the next two chapters. Table 3.6 may help you in deciding on the most appropriate chart for any given set of data.

Table 3.6:   Choosing an appropriate chart

DATA TYPE	PIE CHART	BAR CHART	DOTPLOT	VERTICAL LINE CHART	HISTOGRAM (if grouped)	STEP CHART	OGIVE
Nominal	yes	yes	no	no	no	no	no
Ordinal	no	yes	yes	no	no	yes*	no
Metric discrete	no	yes	yes	yes	yes	yes*	no
Metric continuous	no	no	yes†	no	yes	no	yes*

*Cumulative. †If integer.

4

DESCRIBING DATA FROM ITS DISTRIBUTIONAL SHAPE

Learning objectives

When you have finished this chapter you should be able to:

- *Explain what is meant by the "shape" of a frequency distribution*
- *Sketch and explain negatively skewed, symmetric, and positively skewed distributions*
- *Sketch and explain a bimodal distribution*
- *Interpret the likely shape of a frequency distribution from a frequency table or chart*
- *Sketch and describe a Normal distribution*

The Shape of Things to Come

Both frequency tables and charts, but especially charts, can be used to describe the *shape* of a frequency distribution. For example, are the values fairly evenly spread throughout their possible range? Are most of them concentrated towards the bottom or towards the top of the range? Do the values clump together around any particular value? And so on. Distributional shape can be *broadly* categorised as being left-skewed, right-skewed, symmetric and mound-shaped, or bimodal. Inevitably, distributional shape also influences the choice of the most appropriate method of analysis. One simple way to assess the shape of a frequency distribution is to plot a bar chart, a dotplot, or a histogram, as you saw in Chapter 3.

TWO EXAMPLES OF SHAPE FROM PRACTICE, AND ONE FROM THIN AIR

Symmetric Mound-shaped Distributions

The histogram in Figure 4.1 is from a study into the use of the mammography service by women in the 33 health districts of Ontario, from mid-1990 to end-1991. The investigators were interested in the variation in the use of the mammography service (the utilisation rate is the number of consultations per 1000 women), between women in the age groups 30–39, 40–49, 50–59, and 70+ years. These utilisation rates are plotted with a histogram (actually, this is more like a bar chart than a histogram, with gaps incorrectly appearing between the bars). However, you can see that the distribution is reasonably symmetric and mound-shaped. Note also that for the birthweight data in Table 2.1, SPSS and Minitab provide summary values of: mean = 3644.4g, median = 3614.0g. The similarity of these values also suggests a symmetric shape.

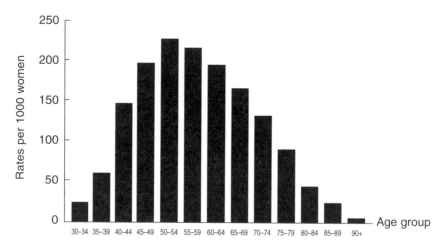

Figure 4.1:   Histogram of mammography utilisations rate (per 1000 women), by broad age group, in 33 health districts in Ontario, 1990–91

Skewed Distributions

Look back at the APACHE II scores in Figure 3.7. As you can see, most of the values lie in the upper end of the distribution with progressively fewer and fewer towards the lower end. Such a distribution is said to be *negatively skewed*.

The histogram in Figure 4.2, showing serum E_2 levels from a study of HRT for osteoporosis prevention, has most of its values in the lower end of the distribution with progressively fewer and fewer towards the upper end. There is a single high-valued outlier. This distribution is *positively skewed*.

Skewness is the primary measure used to describe this asymmetry feature of frequency distributions, and many computer programs will calculate a *skewness coefficient* for you: this varies between –1 (strong negative skew) and +1 (strong positive skew). Calculated values of zero or close to it imply zero skew, but do not necessarily mean that the distribution is symmetric.

Another measure sometimes encountered in descriptions of shape is *kurtosis*. This measures the "peakiness" of the distribution. The kurtosis coefficient varies between –1 (a flattish shape) and +1 (a peaky or pointy shape).

Exercise 4.1

The simple bar chart in Figure 4.3 is from a study describing the development of a new scale to measure psychiatric anxiety, called the "Psychiatric Symptom Frequency" scale (PSF). Describe the shape of the distribution of PSF in terms of symmetry, skewness, etc. Does this chart tell the whole story?

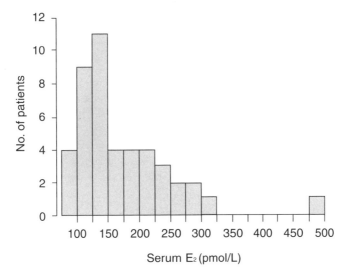

Figure 4.2: Positively skewed frequency curve of the serum E_2 levels in 45 patients in a cross-sectional study of HRT for the prevention of osteoporosis

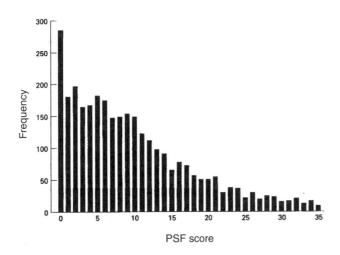

Figure 4.3: Simple bar chart showing the lowest 95% of values of the Psychiatric Symptom Frequency scale (PSF)

Exercise 4.2
Comment on the shapes of the age distributions shown in Table 3.4 for male and female suicide attempters, and later succeeders (you may also want to look at the histograms you drew in Exercise 3.7).

Exercise 4.3
Comment on the shape of the APACHE II scores in Figure 3.6.

Bimodal Distributions

A bimodal distribution is one with two distinct humps. These are less common than the shapes described above, and are often the result of two separate distributions which have not been disentangled. Figure 4.4 shows a hypothetical bimodal distribution of systolic blood pressure. The upper peak could be due to a subgroup of hypertensive patients, but whose presence has not been identified.

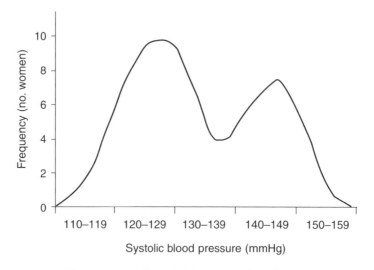

Figure 4.4:   A bimodal frequency distribution

NORMAL-NESS

There is one particular symmetric bell-shaped distribution, known as the *Normal distribution*, which has a special place in the heart of statisticians. Note the capitalised "N", to distinguish this statistical usage from that of the word "normal" meaning usual, ordinary, etc. Because the Normal distribution is by definition symmetric, the mean, median and mode will all have the same value. Many human clinical features are distributed Normally: for example, height, weight, blood pressure, birthweight, and a lot more. The Normal distribution has a very important role to play in what is to come.

An Example from Practice

Figure 4.5 shows a histogram for the distribution of the cord platelet count (10^9/L) in 4382 Finnish infants, from a cross-sectional study into the prevalence and causes of thrombocytopenia in full-term infants.[1] You can see, even without the help of the Normal curve superimposed upon it, that the distribution has a very regular bell-shaped symmetric distribution. In fact this is pretty well as Normal as it gets with real data.

---

[1] Thrombocytopenia is deemed to exist when the cord platelet count is less than 150×10^9/L. It is a risk factor for intraventricular haemorrhage and contributes to the high neurological morbidity in infants affected.

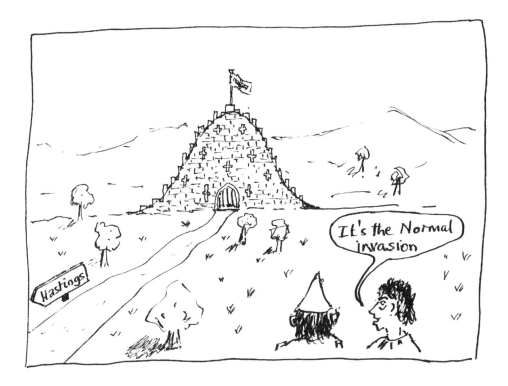

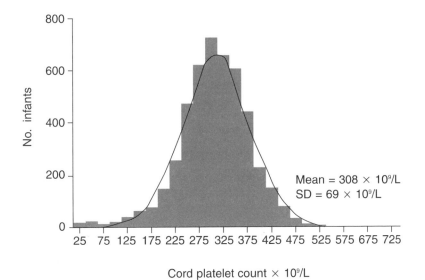

Figure 4.5: A Normal frequency curve superimposed on a histogram of cord platelet count (10^9/L) in 4382 infants

Exercise 4.4

Table 4.1 shows the age distribution of 1299 women in a study into the effectiveness of hysterectomy in relieving adverse symptoms. How would you describe the shape of the age distribution of these women?

Table 4.1: The distribution of age of 1299 women in a cohort study into the effectiveness of hysterectomy in relieving adverse symptoms

AGE (years)	PERCENTAGE FREQUENCY
<30	4.6
30–39	31.6
40–49	47.3
50–59	9.5
60–69	4.4
70+	2.6

OTHER DISTRIBUTIONS

Although the Normal distribution is one of the most important in a health context, you may also encounter others, such as the *binomial* and *Poisson* distributions.

- As an example of the former, suppose you are to choose 20 patients at random from a very large list of patients containing *equal* numbers of males and females. The chance of picking a male patient with each successive pick is thus 1 in 2. The binomial distribution describes the chance of getting any given number of males (or females), from 0 to 20, in your 20 selected patients.
- The Poisson distribution describes the probability of a chosen number of events occurring in a fixed period of time: for example, the probability of some given number of patients arriving at an A&E department in one hour.

Space limitations prevent any further discussion of either of these distributions.

To sum up so far. You have seen that you can describe the principal features of a set of data using tables and charts. A description of the shape of the distribution is also an important part of the picture. In the next chapter you will meet a way of describing data using numeric *summary* values.

5

DESCRIBING DATA WITH NUMERIC SUMMARY VALUES

Learning objectives

When you have finished this chapter you should be able to:

- *Calculate and explain the difference between a percentage and a proportion*
- *Explain what prevalence and incidence are*
- *Explain what a summary measure of location is, and show that you understand the meaning of and the difference between the mode, the median and the mean*
- *Be able to calculate the mode, median and mean for a set of values*
- *Demonstrate that you understand the role of data type and distributional shape in choosing the most appropriate measure of location*
- *Explain what a percentile is, and calculate any given percentile value*
- *Explain what a summary measure of spread is, and show that you understand the difference between, and can calculate, the index of qualitative variation, the range, the interquartile range, and the standard deviation*
- *Show that you can estimate percentile values from an ogive*
- *Demonstrate that you understand the role of data type and distributional shape in choosing the most appropriate measure of spread*
- *Draw a boxplot and explain how it works*
- *Show that you understand the area properties of the Normal distribution and how these relate to standard deviation*

Numbers R Us

There are two features of a set of data which can each be summarised with a single numeric value:

- First, a value around which the data has a tendency to congregate, called a *summary measure of location*.[1]
- Second, a value that measures the degree to which the data is, or is not, spread out, called a *summary measure of spread*.

With these two values you can then compare different sets of data *quantitatively*. Before I discuss these two measures, however, let's look first at a number of other, simpler numeric measures.

---

[1] Also known as a *measure of central tendency*.

NUMBERS, PERCENTAGES AND PROPORTIONS

The simplest numerical summaries of data are numbers—for example, the numbers of males and females, or the numbers of smokers—whatever seems particularly interesting and relevant to a study. In Table 1.2, from the stress/breast cancer study, the authors give the numbers of women with breast cancer (the cases), and the number without breast cancer (the controls). The figures, $n = 106$ and $n = 226$ respectively, are given at the top of their respective columns.

Data may also be summarised by calculating *percentages* or *proportions*.[2] In Table 1.2 the authors give the percentage of subjects who are in each "social class" category. For example, 26% and 32% of the cases and controls, respectively, are in the category "III non-manual".[3] As in this example, it is usually categorical data that is summarised with a value for percentage or proportion.

Exercise 5.1
Using the values in the first row of Table 3.2, calculate the proportion and percentage of men among those subjects who were (a) breast-fed; (b) bottle-fed.

One Other Interesting Fact

Suppose you record some attribute or quality of a study subject by scoring 0 for an absence of the attribute, and 1 for the presence of the attribute. For example, Table 5.1 shows the HIV status (0 = HIV−; 1 = HIV+) of eight intravenous drug-users admitted to an A&E department. The proportion of patients HIV+ (i.e. the proportion of 1s) is 5/8 = 0.625, or 62.5%. Now, if you calculate the *average* of the HIV status column, you get:

$$(1 + 0 + 0 + 1 + 1 + 1 + 0 + 1)/8 = 5/8 = 0.625.$$

In other words the average of a column of 0,1 values is the *proportion* of 1s. We'll use this very useful property later in the book.

Table 5.1:   HIV status of eight subjects: 0 = HIV−, 1 = HIV+

PATIENT	1	2	3	4	5	6	7	8
HIV STATUS	1	0	0	1	1	1	0	1

Prevalence and the Incidence Rate

Data can also be described by providing a summary figure of prevalence or incidence. The *point prevalence* of a disease is the number of *existing* cases in some population at a given time. In practice, however, the *period prevalence* is more often used. It might typically be reported as "the prevalence of genital chlamydia in single women in England in 1996 was 3.1%". This figure will of course include existing cases—i.e. those who contracted the disease before 1996, and still had it, as well as those first getting the disease in 1996.

---

[2] A percentage (%) is just a proportion multiplied by 100.
[3] $(28/106) \times 100 = 26$ and $(72/226) \times 100 = 32$.

The *incidence* or inception rate of a disease is the number of *new* cases occurring per 1000, or per 10,000 (or whatever base is arithmetically appropriate), of the population, during some period of time, usually 12 months. The age-specific referral rates shown in Table 1.1 are another example of incidence rates.

Exercise 5.2
(a) When a group of 890 women were tested for genital chlamydia with a ligase chain reaction test, 23 of the women had a positive response. Assuming the test is always 100% efficient, what is the prevalence of genital chlamydia among women in this group?
(b) Suppose in a certain city there were 10,000 live births in 2002. Ten of the infants died of sudden infant death syndrome. What is the incidence rate for sudden infant death syndrome in this city?

SUMMARY MEASURES OF LOCATION

A summary measure of location, roughly speaking, is that value around which most of the data values tend to congregate or centre. I am going to discuss three measures of location: the mode, the median and the mean. As you will see, the choice of the most appropriate measure depends crucially on the type of data involved. I will summarise which measure(s) you can most appropriately use with which type of data later in the chapter.

The Mode

The *mode* is that category or value which *occurs the most often*. In this sense the mode is a measure of *typical-ness*. The mode is appropriate if your data is categorical (nominal or ordinal), but it *can* be used also with metric discrete data. Metric continuous data is rarely suitable for summarising with the mode, since there may well be no two data values the same—although if the data is in integer form, as age for example often is, the mode could be used.

As an example, the modal Apgar score in Figure 2.1 is 8, this being the category with the highest frequency (of nine infants); i.e. it is the most commonly occurring. Of course you could have calculated the mode from the raw data, but since the frequency table was handy, I used it. In any case, if you are calculating a mode by hand, it's easier to first construct a frequency table.

Exercise 5.3
Determine the modal value or category for: (a) social class for both cases and controls, in the stress and breast cancer study shown in Figure 1.2; (b) level of satisfaction with nursing care, for the data in Figure 2.2; (c) PSF score in Figure 4.3.

The Median

If data is arranged in ascending order of size, the *median* is the middle value, with half of the values equal to or less than it, and half equal to or above it. In other words, the median is a measure of *central-ness*. For example, suppose you had the following data on age (years), for five individuals in ascending order: 30 31 **32** 33   35. The middle value is 32, so the median age for these five people is 32 years.

If you have an *even* number of values, the median is the average of the two values each side of the "middle". So for example, if you have six people with ages of 30 31 **32** **33** 35   36, then the median is the average of 32 and 33, i.e. 32.5 years.

To get a bit technical for a moment (it comes in useful a little later on), if you have n values arranged in order, then the median is the $\frac{1}{2}(n + 1)$th value. In the above example $n = 6$, so $\frac{1}{2}(n + 1) = \frac{1}{2}(6 + 1) = \frac{1}{2}(7) = 3.5$. So the median is the 3.5th value—i.e. half-way between the third value, 32, and the fourth value, 33—or 32.5 years, which is the same result as before.

The median can be used with both ordinal and metric data (both can be arranged in order), but not with nominal data whose ordering is, as you know, arbitrary. One limitation of the median is that it does not use all of the information in the data. In fact apart from the middle value (or two) the rest of the values are ignored. For example, suppose the ages of the above six people were 30 31 32 33 98 99. The median is still 32.5 years!

On the other hand, the median is a *stable* summary measure. In other words, as you have just seen, it is not affected by changes in the values at either end of the distribution (including any outliers).

Exercise 5.4
(a) Determine the median percentage mortality of the 26 ICUs in Table 2.5 (see also Exercise 2.3). (b) From the data in Figure 3.12 and for later successful suicides, determine which age group contains the median age for (i) men, and (ii) women.

The Mean

The *mean*—in everyday speak the *average*—is easily calculated by dividing the sum of the values by the number of values. Note that this calculation requires us to use arithmetic; and since you already know that it is not appropriate to use arithmetic with ordinal values, it follows that you should *not* try to calculate a mean for ordinal data. Obviously, the mean of nominal categorical data has no meaning—after all, what is the average hair colour, or the average sex, of the children in the nit-lotion study which you encountered in Chapter 1? As Spock would say: "It doesn't compute, Captain." This implies that you can only use the mean as your summary measure of location with metric data, whether discrete or continuous.

In contrast to the median, the mean *does* use every sample value, but is consequentially influenced by extreme values (*outliers*). If these are present in the data, the mean will be "dragged" in their direction. This may produce a mean which is not very representative of the general mass of the data. The relative sizes of the mean and the median thus provide a clue about the direction of any skew, as follows:

mean > median = positive skew;
mean < median = negative skew;
mean ≈ median = symmetrical-ish distribution.

Exercise 5.5
Comment on the likely relative sizes of the mean and median in the distributions of (a) serum potassium, and (b) serum E_2, shown in the histograms in Figure 3.10 and Figure 4.2.

Exercise 5.6
Determine the mean percentage mortality in the 26 ICUs in Table 2.5, and compare with the median value you determined in Exercise 5.4(a).

Exercise 5.7
The histogram of red blood cell thioguanine nucleotide concentration (RBCTNC), measured in pmol/8 × 10^8 red blood cells, in 49 children, shown in Figure 5.1, is from a study into the potential causes of high incidence of secondary brain tumours in children after radiotherapy. (a) Using the information in the figure, calculate median and mean RBCTNC for the 49 children. (b) Remove the two outlier values of 3300, and recalculate the mean and median. Compare and comment on the two sets of results.

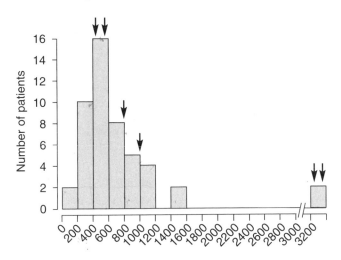

Thioguanine nucleotide concentration
(pmol/8 × 10^8 red blood cells)

Figure 5.1: Histogram of red blood cell thioguanine nucleotide concentration (RBCTNC) before cranial radiotherapy, in 49 children. Arrows show values for six patients who went on to develop secondary brain tumours

Percentiles

Suppose you have birthweights for 1200 infants, which you've put in ascending order. You now identify the birthweight which has 1% of the birthweight values below it (i.e. 12 values) and 99% above it (i.e. 1188 values). This value is known as the *1st percentile*. Similarly, the birthweight which has 2% birthweight values below it and 98% above it is called the *2nd percentile*. You could repeat this process until you reached the 99th percentile, which would have 99% (1188) of birthweight values below it and only 1% (12) above it. In other words the percentile values (or just *"centile values"*) divide the total number of birthweights, or any other set of ordered values, into 100 equal-sized groups.

This makes the median the *50th centile*, since it divides the data values into two equal halves, 50% above the median and 50% below. How then do you determine any particular centile value? Take the example of the 30 birthweights in Table 2.1, which are reproduced below, but now in ascending order, along with their position in the order:

2860	2994	3193	3266	3287	3303	3388	3399	3400	3421
1	2	3	4	5	6	7	8	9	10

3447	3508	3541	3594	3613	3615	3650	3666	3710	3798
11	12	13	14	15	16	17	18	19	20

3800	3886	3896	4006	4010	4090	4094	4200	4206	4490
21	22	23	24	25	26	27	28	29	30

Recall that the median is the $\frac{1}{2}(n + 1)$th value. Now $\frac{1}{2}$ is the same as $50/100$, so this can be rewritten as $(50/100) \times (n + 1)$, bearing in mind that the median is the 50th centile. If you want to determine the 20th centile, the formula becomes $(20/100) \times (n + 1)$. Thus the 20th percentile is the $(20/100) \times (30 + 1)$th value $= 0.2 \times$ 31th value $= 6.2$th value. The sixth value is 3303g and the seventh value is 3388g, a difference of 85g; so the 20th centile is 3303g plus 0.2×85g, which is 3303g + 17g = 3320g.

You might be thinking, this all seems a bit messy, but in practice of course you would use a suitable computer program to calculate these values; both SPSS and Minitab perform these calculations effortlessly.

As well as percentiles, you might also encounter *deciles*, which sub-divide the data values into 10, not 100, equal divisions, and *quintiles*, which sub-divide the values into five equal-sized groups. Collectively, percentiles, deciles and quintiles are called *n-tiles*.

Exercise 5.8
Calculate the 25th and 75th percentiles for the ICU percentage mortality values in Figure 2.5, and explain your results.

Choosing the Most Appropriate Measure

How do you choose the most appropriate measure of location for some given set of data?

- If your data is *nominal*, you can *only* use the *mode*.
- If your data is *ordinal*, the *median* is generally the most appropriate. However, in some circumstances you might want to use the mode.
- If your data is *metric*, use the *mean*—unless you think that the presence of marked skewness and/or outliers will produce a misleading result, or for some particular reason you want a summary measure of centrality, in which case use the median. Remember the median doesn't use all of the information in the data.

I have summarised these choices in Table 5.2. As an illustration of the last point, look again at Figure 3.9 which shows the distribution of the number of measles cases in 37 schools. Not only is this distribution very positively skewed, it has a single high-valued outlier. The median number of measles cases is 1.00, but the mean number is 2.91, almost three times as many! The problem is that the outlier is dragging the mean to the right. Here, the median value of 1 seems to be more generally representative of the data than the mean.

Table 5.2: Choosing an appropriate measure of location

DATA TYPE	MODE	MEDIAN	MEAN
Nominal	yes	no	no
Ordinal	yes	yes	no
Metric discrete	yes	yes, if distribution is markedly skewed	yes
Metric continuous	no	yes, if distribution is markedly skewed	yes

SUMMARY MEASURES OF SPREAD

As well as a summary measure of location, a summary measure of *spread* is also a very handy description of the degree to which the data is dispersed, or not dispersed, across its range. I want to consider four such summary measures here, and once again, as you will see, the choice of an appropriate measure is influenced by the type of data involved.

The Index of Qualitative Variation (IQV)

Summary measures of spread for nominal data appear very rarely in the litera-ture, and as far as I know are just as seldom used. However, in case you ever need such a measure, the *index of qualitative variation* will do the job. It is based on the proportion of values in each category. The more equal these proportions are, the higher the IQV. Unfortunately neither SPSS nor Minitab will compute IQV, so if you ever need to calculate IQV you will have to do it by hand,[4] as follows:

If p_1 is the proportion of values in the first category, p_2 is the proportion in the second, and so on, and if the number of categories is k, then:

$$IQV = [1 - (p_1^2 + p_2^2 + ... + p_k^2)] \times k/(k-1).$$

IQV varies between 0 (all values in one category) and 1 (equal number of values in each category). Look back at Figure 3.1, which shows the number of children, out of a total of 95, assigned to one of four hair colour categories in the nit-lotion study. It's easy enough to calculate the proportions in each category as: $p_1 = 0.158$

---

[4] You may be aware of a computer program that will calculate IQV.

(blonde), p_2 = 0.516 (brown), p_3 = 0.042 (red), and p_4 = 0.284 (dark). With four categories, k = 4, and substituting in the above expression gives us:

$$IQV = [1 - (0.158^2 + 0.516^2 + 0.042^2 + 0.284^2)] \times 4/(4 - 1)$$
$$= (1 - 0.374) \times 1.333 = 0.835.$$

This value is towards the top of the IQV range and indicates a reasonably even division of values across categories. By itself this may not be very helpful. IQV is of more use if you want to compare the spread in *two* or more nominal distributions with equal numbers of categories.

The Range

The range is the distance from the smallest value to the largest. For example, the range of the 30 birthweights in Table 2.1 is from 2860g to 4490g. The range is best written in the form: range = (2860g to 4490g).

Exercise 5.9
What are the ranges for age among those breast-fed and those bottle-fed in Table 3.2?

You can use the range with both ordinal and metric data (both of which can be ordered), but *not* with nominal data. A limitation of the range is that it is an unstable measure—i.e. it is very much effected by the presence of outliers, since of course you use the most extreme values in its calculation. However, sometimes, knowledge of the range may be useful.

The Interquartile Range (IQR)

One solution to the sensitivity of the range to extreme values (outliers) is to chop a quarter of the values off both ends of the distribution, which gets rid of any troublesome outliers, and then measure the range of what's left. This is called the *interquartile range* or IQR. So the IQR measures the spread of the *middle* half or 50% of the values. You can use the interquartile range with both ordinal and metric data.

To calculate the IQR you need first to determine two values: the value which cuts off the bottom 25% of values, known as the *1st quartile* and denoted Q1, and the value which cuts off the top 25% of values, known as the *3rd quartile* and denoted Q3. The IQR is then written as:

IQR = (Q1 to Q3).

I used SPSS and Minitab to calculate the quartile birthweight values in Table 2.1, which are Q1 = 3396.25g and Q3 = 3923.50g. Therefore:

IQR = (3396.25g to 3923.50g).

This result tells you that the middle 50% of infants weighed between 3396.25g and 3923.50g.

An Example from Practice

Table 5.3 describes the baseline characteristics of 56 patients in an investigation into the use of analgesics in the prevention of stump and phantom pain in lower-limb amputation. The "blockade" group of patients ($n = 27$) were given bupivacaine and morphine, the control (comparison) group ($n = 29$), were given an identically administered saline placebo.

Table 5.3   The baseline characteristics of 56 patients in an investigation into the use of analgesics in the prevention of stump and phantom pain in lower-limb amputation

CHARACTERISTICS OF PATIENTS	BLOCKADE GROUP ($n = 27$)	CONTROL GROUP ($n = 29$)
Men/women	15/12	18/11
Mean (SD) age in years	72.8 (13.2)	70.8 (11.4)
Diabetes	10	14
Concurrent treatment because of cardiovascular disease	18	19
Previous stroke	3	2
Previous contralateral amputation	7	3
Median (IQR) pain in week before amputation (VAS, 0–100mm)	51 (23.8–87.8)	44 (25.3–36.8)
Median (IQR) daily opioid consumption at admission (mg)	50 (20–68.8)	30 (5–62.5)
Level of amputation		
Below knee	15	16
Through knee-joint	5	2
Above knee	7	11
Reamputations during follow-up	3	2
Died during follow-up	10	10

As you can see, two variables, "Pain in week before amputation", and "Daily opioid consumption at admission (mg)", were summarised with median and IQR values. Pain was measured using a visual analogue scale (VAS).[5] The VAS produces ordinal data so the mean is not appropriate, and the authors have chosen the median and interquartile range as their summary measures of location and spread. The median level of pain in the blockade group is 51, with an IQR of (23.8 to 87.8).[6]. This means that 25% of this group had a pain level of less than 23.8, and 25% a pain level greater than 87.8. The middle 50% had a pain level between 23.8 and 87.8. I'll return to the opioid consumption variable shortly.

Exercise 5.10
Calculate the IQR for the ICU percentage mortality values in Table 2.5. (You have already calculated the 25th and 75th percentiles in Exercise 5.8.)

---

[5] See Exercise 1.3.
[6] The published table contained a typographical error, recording 87.8 as "8–78".

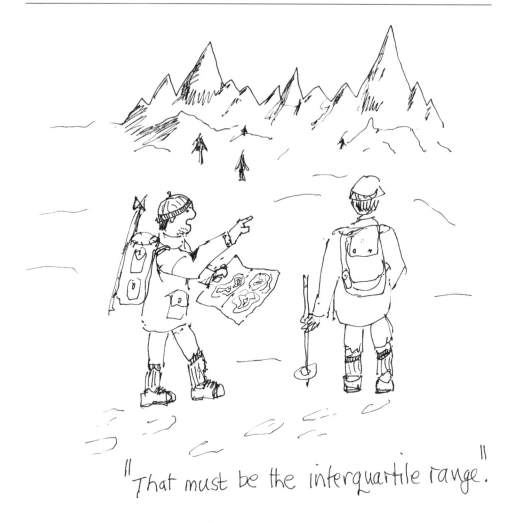

"That must be the interquartile range."

Exercise 5.11
(a) Interpret the median and interquartile range values for pain in the week before amputation for the control group in Table 5.3.

Estimating the Median and Interquartile Range from the Ogive

As I hinted earlier, you can estimate the median and/or the interquartile range from the cumulative frequency curve (the ogive). Look at Figure 5.2 which is the ogive for the cumulative birthweight data shown in Figure 3.12.

If you draw horizontal lines from the values 25%, 50% and 75% on the y axis to the ogive and then down to the x axis, the points of intersection on the x axis will give you estimates of Q1, Q2 (the median), and Q3. These appear to be about 3400g, 3600g and 3900g. So if you happen to have an ogive handy, these approximations

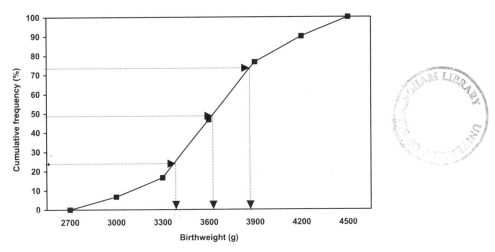

Figure 5.2: Using the relative cumulative frequency curve (or ogive) of birthweight to estimate the median and interquartile range values (note that this *should* be a smooth curve)

can be helpful. Notice that I plotted *percentage* cumulative frequency because it makes it easier to find the 25%, 50% and 75% values on the y axis.

You can also use the ogive to answer questions like "What percentage of infants weighed less than say 4000g?" The answer is that a value of 4000g on the x axis produces a value of 80% for cumulative frequency on the y axis.

Exercise 5.12
Estimate the median and IQR for total blood cholesterol for the control group from the ogive in Figure 3.13.

The Boxplot

I promised in Chapter 3 to introduce the *boxplot*, but we needed to examine the median and interquartile range first. Boxplots provide a graphical summary of the three quartile values, the minimum and maximum values, and any outliers. A boxplot is usually plotted with value on the vertical axis, and like the pie chart the boxplot can represent only one variable at a time, but a number of boxplots can be set alongside each other. Both SPSS and Minitab will draw boxplots, but unfortunately not Word's or Excel's chart tool.

An Example from Practice

Figure 5.3 is from the same study as Figure 4.1, into the use of the mammography service in the 33 health districts of Ontario, between mid-1990 and end-1991. The investigators were interested in the variation in the mammography utilisation rate within the health districts and between age groups. They supplemented their results with the boxplots shown in the figure, for the age groups 30–39, 40–49, 50–69, and 70+ years. The vertical axis is the mammography utilisation rate (visits per 1000 women), in the 33 health

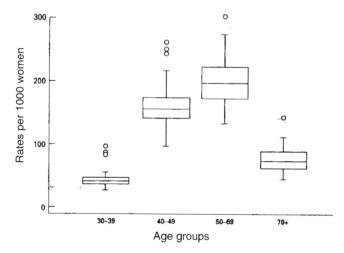

Figure 5.3: Boxplots of the rate of use of mammography services in 33 health districts in Ontario, from a cross-sectional study into the use of the mammography service between mid-1990 and end-1991

districts. Outliers are denoted by the small open circles. You can interpret the boxplots as follows (focussing on the 50–59 age group).

The bottom end of the lower "whisker" (the line sticking out of the bottom of the box) corresponds to the minimum rate—about 125 visits per 1000 women aged 50–69, across the 33 health districts. The bottom of the box is the 1st quartile value, Q1—about 175 per 1000 women (so 25% of health districts had a utilisation rate less than 175). The line inside the box (it won't always be half-way up) is the median, Q2. So in 50% of health districts, women aged 50–69 had a utilisation rate of less than about 200 consultations, 50% more than 200. The top of the box is the third quartile, Q3—about 225 consultations per 1000 women. This means that 25% of the health districts have a utilisation rate above 225. The top end of the upper whisker is the maximum mammography utilisation rate—about 275 consulta-tions per 1000 women.

There is one outlier. One of the health districts reported a utilisation rate of about 300 per 1000 women.[7] The more asymmetric the distributional shape, the further away from the middle of the box is the median line—closer to the top of the box with negative skew, or to the bottom of the box with positive skew.

Exercise 5.13
Sketch the boxplot for the percentage mortality in ICUs shown in Table 2.5 (note that you have already calculated the median and IQR values in Exercises 5.4 and 5.10.) What can you glean from the boxplot about the shape of the distribution of the ICU percentage mortality rate?

Exercise 5.14
The boxplots in Figure 5.4 are from a study to investigate a new technique of laparoscopic lymphadenectomy for the treatment of cervical cancer, and show the para-

---

[7] Outliers are defined in various ways by different computer programs. One definition is any value which lies more than two box heights from the median.

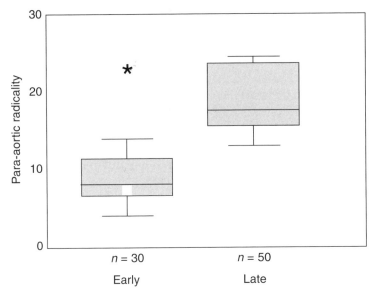

Figure 5.4: Boxplots from a study to investigate a new technique of laparoscopic lymphadenectomy for treatment of cervical cancer, showing the para-aortic radicality, in two groups of women, one group treated early in the study, the second group treated late in the study. Higher scores indicate more successful treatment

aortic radicality in two groups of women: one group treated early in the study, and one four years later at the end of the study. The objective was to determine whether more experience with the procedure would lead to a greater degree of radicality (i.e. a more clinically successful lymphadenectomy). What do the two boxplots tell you?

Standard Deviation

One problem with the range is that it is too sensitive to outliers. A limitation of the interquartile range is that (like the median) it doesn't use all of the information in the data, loosing the top and bottom quarter of the values. One summary measure of spread that does use all of the information in the data is the *standard deviation* (abbreviated to SD, or sd).

The standard deviation is based on the idea of summarising the spread in a set of data by measuring *the average distance of all the data values from the mean value*. Clearly, the smaller this average distance is, the narrower the spread, and vice versa.

To illustrate, suppose you have the following parity values for a group of five women: 1   3   5   7   9. Mean parity = $(1 + 3 + 5 + 7 + 9)/5 = 25/5 = 5$. The distance of each value from this mean of 5 is:

$(5 - 1) = 4; (5 - 3) = 2; (5 - 5) = 0; (7 - 5) = 2; (9 - 5) = 4.$

The average distance from the mean is therefore $(4 + 2 + 0 + 2 + 4)/5 = 2.4$. So the values are, on average, 2.4 from the mean.

Consider now the following parity data for a second group of women: 3 4 5 6 7. The spread of parity values in this second group is narrower than for the first group, so let's see how this is reflected in their average distance from their mean. Following the above procedure, the average distance from the mean for this second group is only 1.2, half of that for the first group, so a measure of average distance from the mean *does* capture difference in spreads.

In truth, calculation of standard deviation is a little more complicated than this, but based on this same idea. I cheated above by treating all of the difference-from-mean terms as being positive, when of course those less than the mean will be negative. The problem is that negative and positive differences *always* cancel each other out (they always sum to zero), but the basic idea is too good to abandon. The following procedure overcomes the cancelling problem and gives a measure of the average distance from the mean which works:

- Subtract the mean from each of the n values in the sample, to give the difference values.
- Square each of these differences.
- Add these squared values together (called the "sum of squares")
- Divide the sum of squares by 1 less than the sample size. That is, divide by $(n-1)$.[8]
- Take the square-root.

This calculation is very tedious by hand, especially if you have a lot of values, so again you will want to use your computer. It's important to note that *the standard deviation should only be only be used with metric data*, because, as you saw in Chapter 1, it is not appropriate to apply arithmetic operations to nominal or ordinal data (and calculation of the mean and standard deviation require these).

Exercise 5.15

In Figure 4.5, the authors tell us that the mean cord platelet count is $306 \times 10^9/L$, and the standard deviation is $69 \times 10^9/L$ (notice the two measures have the same units).[9] Explain what this SD value means.

An Example from Practice

In Figure 5.3, the analgesic/amputation pain study, the authors summarise the age of the patients in the study with the mean and standard deviation. As you can see, mean age in the blockade group is 72.8 years, less than that of the control group's 70.8 years. The spread of ages in the blockade group is wider than in the control group, 13.2 years compared with 11.4 years.

The authors could also have used the mean and standard deviation for daily opioid consumption (mg) since this is a metric variable. Instead they chose to use the median and IQR, and there are a number of reasons why they may have made this choice. First, the data may be noticeably skewed and/or contained outliers, perhaps making the mean a

---

[8] If we divide by n, as we normally would to find a mean, we get a result which is slightly too small. Dividing by $(n-1)$ adjusts for this. Technically, the sample's SD is said to be a biased estimator of the population's SD. See Chapter 7 for the meaning of "sample" and "population".
[9] 10^9 means 1000 million.

little too unrepresentative of the general mass of data. Alternatively the investigators may have specifically wanted a summary measure of central-ness, which the median provides. Third, they may have felt that asking people to recall their opioid consumption last week was likely to lead to fuzzy, imprecise values, and so have preferred to treat them as if they were ordinal.

Exercise 5.16
Calculate and interpret the standard deviation for the ICU percentage mortality values in Table 2.5. (You have already calculated the mean percentage mortality in Exercise 5.6.) I would hesitate to do this without a computer or a calculator with a standard deviation function!

Summary

With nominal data you could use the index of qualitative variation as a summary measure of spread. With ordinal data you could use either the range or the interquartile range, but the standard deviation is not appropriate because of the non-numeric nature of ordinal data. With metric data you could use either the standard deviation, which uses all of the information in the data, or the interquartile range. Use the latter if the distribution is skewed, and/or you have already selected the median as your preferred measure of location. Don't mix-and-match these measures: standard deviation goes with the mean, and IQR goes with the median. Table 5.4 summarises the appropriateness of the various measures of dispersion.

Table 5.4   Choosing an appropriate measure of spread

DATA TYPE	RANGE	INTERQUARTILE RANGE	STANDARD DEVIATION
Nominal	no	no	no
Ordinal	yes	yes	no
Metric	yes	yes	yes

STANDARD DEVIATION AND THE NORMAL DISTRIBUTION

If you are working with metric data which is distributed Normally, the standard deviation has one very useful property, which relates to the percentage of data between certain values. These *area properties*, are illustrated in Figure 5.5 for the birthweight data in Table 2.1 (assumed to be Normal). I used Minitab to calculate that the mean birthweight was 3644g with a standard deviation of 377g. In other words:

- About 67% of the birthweights will lie within *one* standard deviation either side of the mean; that is, from 3644g – 377g to 3644g + 377g, which is from 3267g to 4021g.
- About 95% of the birthweights will lie within *two* standard deviations either side of the mean; that is, from 3644g – 754g to 3644g + 754g, which is from 2890g to 4398g.

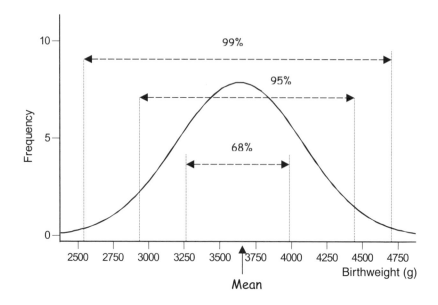

Figure 5.5: Area properties of the Normal distribution illustrated with the birthweight data in Table 2.1

- About 99% of the birthweights will lie within *three* standard deviations either side of the mean; that is, from 3644g – 1131g to 3644g + 1131g, which is from 2513g to 4775g.

The usefulness of these properties is twofold. First, if you have some data which you know is Normally distributed, and you also know the values of the mean and standard deviation, then you can make statements such as "I know that 95% of the values must lie within so-and-so and so-and-so".

Second, if you have some data and you are not sure whether or not it is Normally distributed, the area properties might at least help you to *rule out* a Normal distribution. As an example, suppose you have some data on age, and you know the mean is 40 years and the standard deviation is 15 years. Now if the data *is* Normally distributed you should be able to fit three standard deviations either side of the mean. But three standard deviations below the mean takes you to (40 – 3 × 15) = –5 years, an impossible value; so age in this example cannot be Normally distributed.

In real life, even if the variable you're measuring is Normally distributed, your data is unlikely to capture this exactly. You will probably have to settle for approximately Normally distributed. However, the further from Normality, the greater the approximation in the area properties.

An Example from Practice

To illustrate the usefulness of the Normal area properties, look again at the histogram of the cord platelet count for 4382 infants in Figure 4.5, which appears to be reasonably Normal, and has a mean of 306×10^9/L, and a standard deviation of 69×10^9/L. You can therefore say that about two-thirds (67%) of the infants (i.e. 2966) had a cord platelet count between $306 - 69$ and $306 + 69$, which is between 237 and 375×10^9/L.

Exercise 5.17

Table 5.5 is from a cross-over study of the effectiveness of lisinopril as a prophylactic for acute migraine, in which 47 patients were given the lisinopril and a placebo. Outcome measures included "Hours with headache", "Days with headache", and "Days with migraine", all metric continuous variables. The mean and standard deviation for each of these variables is shown in the table. Do you think they can be Normally or symmetrically distributed? Explain your answer.

Table 5.5 Output measures from a cross-over study of the effectiveness of lisinopril as a prophylactic for acute migraine. Figures are means (SD)

	LISINOPRIL	PLACEBO	MEAN % REDUCTION (95% CI)
Primary efficacy parameter			
Hours with headache	129 (125)	162 (142)	20 (5 to 36)
Days with headache	19.7 (14)	23.7 (11)	17 (5 to 30)
Days with migraine	14.5 (11)	18.5 (10)	21 (9 to 34)
Secondary efficacy parameter			
Headache severity index	297 (325)	370 (310)	20 (3 to 37)
Triptan doses	15.7 (15)	20.2 (17)	22 (7 to 38)
Doses of analgesics	14.5 (23)	16.2 (20)	11 (−16 to 37)
Days with sick leave	2.30 (4.32)	2.09 (2.50)	−10 (−64 to 37)
Bodily pain*	63.7 (29)	53.8 (23)	−18 (−35 to −1)
General health*	73.6 (20)	74.1 (21)	1 (−6 to 7)
Vitality*	61.1 (24)	58.2 (21)	−5 (−18 to 8)
Social functioning*	81.4 (25)	79.5 (23)	−2 (−11 to 6)

*From SF36

TRANSFORMING DATA

Later in the book you will meet some procedures which require that the data involved must be Normally distributed. But what if your data is not Normal? Happily some non-Normal data can be *transformed* to make the distribution reasonably Normal (or at least more Normal than it was to start with). The commonest approach with positively skewed data is to take the *logarithm* of the data (either to base 10 or base e). Other possibilities include taking the square-root or the reciprocal, but it's really a question of trial and error, comparing histograms of the original and transformed data after each transformation is tried. Whatever transformation you use, you will usually have to "back-transform" your final result to return it to its original units (and for it to make sense).

An Example from Practice

Figure 5.6 shows histograms for the original and transformed data on the weight (kg) of 685 women in a diet and health cohort study. The original data is positively skewed. If we transform the data by taking natural logs (logs to the base e), you can see that the transformed data has a more Normal-ish shape.

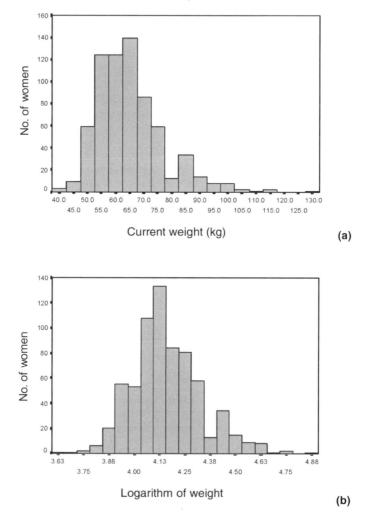

Current weight (kg)   (a)

Logarithm of weight   (b)

Figure 5.6: The effect of applying a logarithmic transformation on the shape of the distribution of the weight of 658 women

In Part II, I have discussed ways of describing data—with tables, with charts, from its shape, and with numeric summary measures. Collectively these various procedures are labelled *descriptive statistics*. However, in all of the above, I assumed that you already had the data which you were describing, and I said nothing about how you might collect the data in the first place. This is the question I will address in the following chapter.

III

GETTING THE DATA

6

DOING IT RIGHT FIRST TIME: DESIGNING A STUDY

Learning objectives

When you have finished this chapter you should be able to:

- *Explain why it is important for a sample to be as representative as possible of the population from which it is taken*
- *Define a random sample*
- *Outline the process of taking stratified, systematic, multistage, cluster, and convenience samples*
- *Explain the difference between observational and experimental studies*
- *Explain the difference between matched and independent groups*
- *Briefly describe case series, cross-section, cohort, and case–control studies*
- *Outline the principal advantages and shortcomings of each of these types of design*
- *Explain the problem of confounding*
- *Outline the general idea of the clinical trial*
- *Explain the concept of randomisation and why it is important, and demonstrate that you can use a random number table to perform a simple block randomisation*
- *Describe the concept of blinding and what it is intended to achieve*
- *Outline and compare the design of the parallel, and cross-over, randomised controlled trials, and summarise their respective advantages and shortcomings*
- *Explain what intention to treat means*
- *Be able to choose an appropriate study design to answer some given research question*

Hey Ho! Hey Ho! It's Off to Work We Go

The genesis of any investigation is a question: "Is exercise an effective treatment for depression?" "What proportion of elderly patients have pressure sores?" "Is a new drug better at reducing hypertension than an existing drug?" And so on. In conjunction with your question you will want to define exactly who your *target* population is, and which group of individuals is in practice actually available, the *study* population (if the two are not the same).

Along with a well-defined question comes a well-defined *outcome measure*. In the exercise and depression question, your outcome measure might be the Beck

Depression Inventory (BDI),[1] and you would want to see whether exercise reduces the *median* BDI score (since this is an ordinal variable). In the two other questions, you might choose the *proportion* of patients with pressure sores, and *mean* blood pressure, respectively.

Now you can turn to the problem of getting the data in the form which will best help to answer your question. You will have to take a sample from your population, and most important of all, a sample which is as *representative* of your population as you can make it. To describe how this might be achieved, I need to discuss two things: first, some ways in which data can be collected from a population; and second, the idea of *study design*, a systematic approach to sample taking and data collection, which offers a clearly defined procedure for organising and conducting studies in a number of different circumstances.

TYPES OF SAMPLE
The Random Sample

Above all you want a *representative* sample. If your target population consists of twice as many men as women, and you end up with a sample with twice as many women as men, any conclusions you draw are likely to be, at least, misleading. The most representative sample of all is a *random sample*. A truly random sample is the "gold standard"—unfortunately rarely if ever achieved in practice. For a sample to be truly random, every member of the population must have an equal chance of being picked for the sample.

However, getting a random sample in the real world is not easy! Take the genital chlamydia example in the previous chapter. If your defined population is all women aged 16+ living in the UK, you would need to know the name and address of every such woman,[2] so that you could write each name on a piece of paper, throw them into a very large hat, and then pick out however many you wanted for your sample. Put crudely. Of course this is not possible, it rarely is.

Systematic Sampling

Since you can't access every 16+ woman in the UK, perhaps you could take as your population all of the women who have attended, during the past 12 months, the well-women clinics attached to the five health centres in your city. These women are all routinely tested for genital chlamydia as part of a general health check. You decide that a sample of 500 women will be big enough (I will return to the question of what is a big enough sample later). Suppose you find that there are 8000 such patients' records in total, and you decide to take every sixteenth record, which will give you 500 records in total. This is a *systematic sample*.

Provided that the list of 8000 records doesn't have some quirky underlying structure which effects every sixteenth person on it, and provided that a sample of 500

---

[1] The BDI is a 30-question questionnaire split into two halves. The patient completes the first 15 questions, the health carer the second 15 questions. Higher scores indicate greater levels of depression.
[2] A comprehensive list like this is called a *sampling frame*.

is big enough to detect a condition which might occur infrequently, the sample should be reasonably representative—*but* representative of the woman attending your five clinics, and not necessarily representative of the entire 16+ female population of the UK. Notice that to take a systemic sample you need a sampling frame.

Stratified Sampling

Suppose you have a particular interest in the occurrence of genital chlamydia in women from some ethnic minority, who you know account for only 10% of your population. To ensure that these women are represented in adequate numbers in your sample (around 10% of the sample), you could separate out the ethnic minority women's records first and then take every sixteenth record from both groups, until you've got 50 from the minority group and 450 from the rest. This process, of stratifying a population before you sample each strata separately, is known as *stratified sampling*. Again you need a sampling frame for this procedure.

Cluster and Multistage Sampling

You could expand your population to include all of the well-women clinics in your health authority; let's say there are 30 clinics. You could then take a random sample of five clinics from these 30, and your subjects would then be *all* of the women in these selected clinics. This approach is known as *cluster sampling*. An alternative approach would be to take a random selection from the 30 clinics and then take a random selection of patients in those clinics. This is *multistage sampling*, an example of which is given below. A sampling frame is not necessary for this method of sampling.

Convenience Sampling

Finally, one approach to the sampling problem is to take as your sample those subjects who are *conveniently* to hand: perhaps the last 100 patients to attend a certain clinic, or all of those patients who attended during the past 12 months. The attraction of convenience sampling is that it is just that, convenient. One obvious problem with this approach is that it is questionable what population such a sample is representative of. In truth, it is extremely difficult to take anything like a true random sample in the healthcare arena. The practical and ethical difficulties associated with such a process are simply too great.

TYPES OF STUDY

Study design divides into two main types, which can be classified in a number of different ways. For example:

- observational versus experimental studies
- or prospective versus retrospective studies
- or longitudinal versus cross-sectional studies.

I am going to use the first classification, although I will explain the other terms on the way. Broadly speaking, an *observational* study is one in which you *actively* observe the subjects involved, perhaps asking questions, or taking some measurements, but you don't control, change, or affect in any way their treatment or care. I will discuss a number of types of observational study designs. An *experimental* study, on the other hand, does involve *active* intervention in the selection, treatment and care of subjects.

OBSERVATIONAL STUDIES

There are four principal types of observational study:

- case-series studies
- cross-section studies
- cohort studies
- case-control studies.

Case-series Studies

A health carer may see a series of patients (cases) with similar but unusual symptoms or outcomes, find something interesting and write it up as a study. This is a *case series*.

An Example from Practice

In 1981 a drug technician at the Centre for Disease Control in the USA noticed an unusually high number of requests for the drug pentamidine, used to treat *Pneumocystis carinii* pneumonia (PCP). This led to a scientific report, a case series study, of PCP occurring unusually in five gay men in Los Angeles. At the same time a similar outbreak of Kaposi's sarcoma (previously rare except in elderly men) in a small number of young gay men in New York also began to raise questions. These events signalled the arrival of HIV in the USA. In the same way, new variant CJD was also first suspected from an unusual series of deaths of young people in the UK, from an apparent dementia-like illness, a disease normally associated with the elderly. Case-series studies often point to a need for further investigations, as in both of these quoted examples.

Cross-section Studies

A cross-section study aims to take a "snapshot" of some situation at some particular point in time, so data from each subject in the study is collected only once.

An Example from Practice

The following extract is from a cross-section study carried out in 1993 on 2542 rural Chinese subjects, into the relationship between body mass index (BMI)[3] and cardiovascular disease (first paragraph). The population of this region of China was about six million, and the 2542 individuals included in the sample were selected using a two-stage sampling process, as the second paragraph explains. Each subject was then interviewed and the necessary measurements were taken (third paragraph).

> The metabolic consequences of obesity are well-documented in Western populations. However, limited data are available on the association between body mass index and cardiovascular risk factors in developing countries. A total of 2542 subjects aged 20–70 years from a rural area of Anqing, China, participated in a cross-sectional survey, and 1610 provided blood samples in 1993. Mean BMI (kg/m^2) was 20.7 for men and 20.9 for women. . . .
>
> These participants were selected from 20 townships in four counties based on a two-stage sampling approach. The sampling unit [was] a village in the first stage and a nuclear family in the second stage, based on the following criteria: (1) both parents alive; and (2) at least two children in the family. We limited the analysis to 2542 participants aged 20 years or older from 776 families. . . .
>
> The survey team was made up of locally hired interviewers fluent in the dialect of the region and faculty members from Anqing Medical University. Local officials and health centers arranged for the interviews and measurements to take place at the central office at times convenient to the participants. Trained interviewers administered questionnaires to gather information on each participant's date of birth, occupation, education level, current cigarette smoking, and alcohol use. Anthropometric measurements, including height and weight, were taken using standard protocols, with subjects not wearing shoes or outer wear. BMI was calculated as weight (kg)/height (m^2). Blood pressure measurements were obtained by trained nurses after subjects had been seated for 10 minutes, by using a mercury manometer and appropriately sized cuffs, according to standard protocols.

Note that there is no intervention by the researchers into any aspect of the subjects' care or treatment (lifestyle advice, for example)—the observers only take measurements, ask some questions, or study records. The results showed that subjects in the sample with higher body mass index values were also likely to have higher blood pressures. The researchers might reasonably claim that this link would also exist in the province's population of 6 million—that's their inference—but the truth of this would depend on how representative the sample was of the whole Anqing population. Whether or not the finding could be extended to the rest of the diverse Chinese population is questionable.

As in many cross-section studies, the researchers in China were trying to uncover a possible link between two (or more) variables, here higher body mass indexes and hypertension. However, a weakness of a cross-section study is that it does not reveal whether a higher BMI leads to higher blood pressures (more strain on the heart, for example), or whether higher blood pressures lead to higher BMI (maybe higher blood pressures effect appetite); it simply establishes some sort of association. I'll return to this "cause and effect" problem shortly, and the "association" question later in the book.

---

[3] Body mass index, used to measure obesity, is equal to a person's weight (kg) divided by their height squared (m)^2. A BMI of between 20 and 25 is considered normal, 25–30 indicates a degree of obesity. Higher scores indicate greater levels of obesity.

A further limitation of the cross-section design is that it is not particularly helpful if the condition being investigated is rare. If, for example, only 0.1% of a population has some particular disease, then a very large sample would have to be taken to produce any worthwhile findings—too small a sample might lead you to conclude that nobody in the population had the disease!

Rather than investigate possible connections, some cross-section studies are more limited in scope and aim only to *describe* some existing state of affairs, such as the prevalence of some condition—for example, the percentage of 16+ individuals in the UK who have taken ecstasy. Only one measurement is taken from each person: have they ever used ecstasy, yes or no? Since this is the only variable measured, no link with any other variable can be explored. Finally, cross-section studies which aim to uncover attitudes, opinions or behaviours are often referred to as *surveys*—for example, the views of clinical staff towards having patients' relatives in A&E trauma rooms.

Cohort Studies: From Here to Eternity

A *cohort study*, also known as a *follow-up*, *prospective* or *longitudinal* study, is one in which a group of individuals, the cohort, is followed "forward" in time. Measurement on the subjects will take place more than once, certainly at the beginning and end of the study, but interim measurements are also possible. Note that "forward" doesn't necessarily mean from *today*, although *prospective* cohort studies *do* follow subjects forward from the time the study is initiated.

A well-known prospective cohort study was that conducted by Doll and Hill into a possible connection between mortality and cigarette smoking. They recruited about 60% of the doctors in the UK, determined their age and smoking status (among other things), and then followed them up over the ensuing years, recording deaths as they arose. Very quickly the data began to show significantly higher mortality among doctors who smoked. The authors would clearly like to infer that this connection was true among all doctors, and also perhaps among the general population. A sample which captures 60% of any population is probably going to be fairly representative, unless of course the 40% not participating were significantly different from the participants. Whether a sample of doctors is also representative of the population at large is more problematic.

In some cohort studies, the data may be collected from existing historical records, and follow subjects from some time starting in the past, as the following example demonstrates.

An Example from Practice

An investigation of the relationship between weight in infancy and the prevalence of coronary heart disease (CHD) in adult life used a sample of 290 men born between 1911 and 1930, and living in Hertfordshire, whose birthweights and weights at one year were on record. In 1994 various measurements were made on the 290 men, including the presence or not of CHD. So "forward" here means forward from 1911 to 1930.

The researchers found that 42 of the 290 men had CHD, a ratio (prevalence) of 14%, but weight at birth was not influential on adult CHD. However, men who weighed 18lb (8.2kg) or less at *one year old* had almost twice the risk of CHD than men who weighed more than 18lb. This of course is only the sample evidence. Whether this finding applies to the population of *all* men born in Hertfordshire during this period, or today, or indeed in the UK, depends on how representative this sample is of either of these populations.

Table 6.1 shows how you can express this cohort study in the form of a contingency table (see Chapter 2). You group the individuals according to their exposure or not to the risk (in this case weighing 18lb or less at one year), and use these groups to form the columns of the table. The rows identify the presence or otherwise of the outcome, CHD.

Table 6.1   Cohort study of the connection between weight at one year and its effect on the presence of CHD in adult life, expressed in the form of a contingency table

OUTCOME: HAS CHD	GROUP BY EXPOSURE TO RISK FACTOR (weighed ≤18lb at 1 year)		Totals
	Yes	No	Totals
Yes	4	38	42
No	11	237	248
Totals	15	275	290

Clearly this design does suggest (but certainly does not prove) a cause and effect—the effect of low weight at one year seems to cause coronary heart disease in adult life.

Cohort studies suffer a number of drawbacks, among which are the following:

- First, selection of a sample of appropriate subjects may cause difficulties. If subjects are chosen using a convenience sample (see above), attendees at a special clinic for example, then the outcomes for these individuals may be different from those in the general population. But population-based sampling is itself difficult as you saw above.
- Second, if the condition is rare in the population—i.e. has low prevalence—it may require a very large cohort to capture enough cases to make the exercise worthwhile.
- Third, the subjects will have to be followed-up for a long time, possibly many years, before any worthwhile results are obtained. This can be expensive as well as frustrating, and not good if a quick answer is needed.
- Fourth, this long time-period allows for considerable losses as subjects drop out for a variety of reasons—they move away, they die from unrelated causes, and so on.
- Fifth, over a long period a significant proportion of the subjects may change their habits, quit smoking for example, or take up regular exercise. However, this problem can be monitored with frequent checks of the state of the cohort.

Finally, note again that the selection of the groups in a cohort study is based on *whether individuals have or have not been exposed to the risk factor*, for example weighing less than 18lb at one year, or smoking.

Case–Control Studies: Back to the Future

A number of the limitations of the cohort design are addressed by the case–control design, although it is itself far from perfect, as you will see. In a cohort study a *single group* of subjects are divided as to whether they are exposed to a particular risk or not (for example, being a cigarette smoker), and then followed-up to see whether they develop a condition of interest (lung cancer or stroke, for example).

In contrast, in a case–control study (also known as a *longitudinal* or *retrospective* study) the groups are selected on the basis of whether individuals have some particular outcome, say lung cancer. So one group consists of individuals who have lung cancer: these are the *cases*. The second group, the *controls*, is then selected so that they are as similar to the cases as possible (same age and sex mix, same employment history, for example), except that they do *not* have lung cancer. Individuals in both groups are then questioned about past smoking habits. It was the outcome from such a case–control study by Doll and Hill which led them to conduct the later cohort study referred to above. Before I discuss the case–control design in more detail, there are a couple of important ideas to be dealt with.

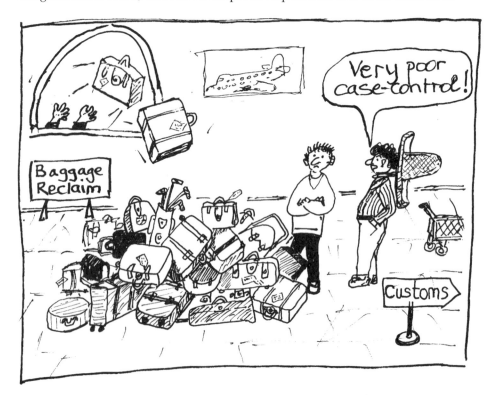

Confounding

You may wonder why we want to ensure that the cases and controls are broadly similar (on age and sex if nothing else). The reason is that it would be very difficult to identify, say, smoking as a risk factor for lung cancer in the cases if these were on average twice as old as the controls—who is to say that it is not increased age that causes the increased risk of lung cancer, not cigarette smoking? But if both groups have much the same age structure (ideally if they are all the *same* age), then any age effect is cancelled out. Similar arguments apply to sex and possibly to other relevant variables, depending on the setting of the research. A variable such as this, which blurs the true nature of the connection between two other variables, say smoking and lung cancer, is known as a *confounder*.

To be a confounder, a variable (say, age), must be associated with *both* the risk factor (smoking) *and* the outcome of interest (lung cancer). People seem to smoke less as they get older, so that's a connection, and the prevalence of lung cancer is greater in older populations, so that's a connection. Similar arguments can be made for sex. So age and sex both qualify as potential confounders, and often are! I'll have more to say about confounding later in the book. When we allow for the effects of possible confounders we are said to be *controlling* or *adjusting*. Results that are based on unadjusted data are said to be "crude" results.

Matching

How we match cases and controls divides case–control studies into two types: the matched and unmatched designs. If each control is *individually* paired, person-to-person, with a case, this is a *matched* case–control design. However, if no attempt is made to match controls—i.e. if they are picked *independently* of the cases, or if the controls are only *broadly* matched (for example, the same broad *mix* of ages, same proportions of males and females, etc. (which is known as *frequency matching*)—then this is an *unmatched* case–control design. The question of whether two sets of data are matched or independent will come up again later, and is a key consideration in the appropriateness of many of the analytic methods we have yet to discuss.

With individuals matched person-to person, you have matched or paired data, which means that the groups of cases and controls are necessarily the same size. Otherwise the matched design has the same underlying principle as the un-matched design. With individual matching the problem of confounding variables is much reduced. However, one practical difficulty is that it is sometimes quite hard to find a suitable control subject to match each case subject on anything more than age and sex.

An Example from Practice

Unmatched case–control design

The following extract, from a frequency-matched case–control study into the possible connection between lifelong exercise and stroke, describes the selection of the case and control subjects.

> Between 1 October 1989 and 30 September 1990 we recruited men and women who had just had their first stroke and were aged 35–74. The patients were assessed by one of us using the standard criteria (for stroke) of the World Health Organization.
>
> Control subjects were randomly selected from the general practice population to broadly match the distribution of age and sex among the patients with stroke (frequency matching). All

those on the register of the 11 participating practices aged 35–74 were eligible for inclusion. The controls were each sent a letter signed by their general practitioner, which was followed up by a telephone call or visit to arrange an appointment for assessment, usually at their practice surgery.

The researchers came up with 125 cases with stroke and 198 controls, broadly matched by age and sex. Notice that the numbers of cases and controls need not be the same (and usually aren't). All subjects (or relatives if necessary) were interviewed and asked about their history (or not) of regular vigorous exercise at various times in the past. Table 6.2 shows the results for those subjects who had and had not taken exercise when they were between the ages of 15 and 25.

Table 6.2 Results from the exercise and stroke unmatched case–control study for those subjects who had and had not exercised between the ages of 15 and 25

RISK FACTOR	GROUP BY OUTCOME (e.g. stroke)	
Exercise aged 15–25	Case	Controls
Yes	55	130
No	70	68

In contrast to a cohort study, in case–control studies you group the subjects by "has outcome (e.g. disease) or not", and this grouping forms the columns. The rows are defined by whether or not subjects were exposed to the risk factor. From these results you can calculate (you'll see how later) that among those who had had a stroke, the chance that they had exercised in their youth was only about half the chance that somebody without a stroke had exercised. Notice that Table 6.2 is not a contingency table because you now have more than one group, the cases and the controls.

An Example from Practice

Matched case–control studies

The following extract is an account of the matching criteria in a 1989 matched case–control study to investigate the hypothesis that significantly stressful life events was a contributory factor in the relapse of breast cancer in women. The authors matched each case with a control on a large number of criteria. They were able to do this because they had a very large number of subjects in their database.

The matching of the women who had a relapse with their controls was performed by computer searches of the database at the clinical oncology unit, Guy's Hospital, which contains clinical, pathological, and demographic information on all women with breast cancer who have attended the unit. The cases and controls were matched in pairs for the main physical and pathological factors known to be prognostic in breast cancer. These included type of operation, whether or not the patient had received adjuvant chemotherapy, menopausal state, affected lymph nodes, tumour size, and histological type of tumour. The cases and controls were then also matched for date of operation and those sociodemographic variables that influence the frequency of life events in the general population.

Comparing Cohort and Case–Control Designs

The case–control design has a number of advantages over the cohort study.

- First, with a cohort study, as you saw above, rare conditions require large samples, but with a case–control study the availability of potential cases is much greater, and sample size can be smaller. Cases will often be selected from patients attending particular clinics, for example.
- Second, case–control studies are cheaper and easier to conduct.
- Third, they give results much more quickly.

But they do have a number of problems, foremost among which is the selection of suitable control subjects. You want subjects who, apart from not having the condition in question, are otherwise similar to the cases. But such individuals are often not easily found. Controls are usually sought either from the general population (and we've seen how difficult that can be), or from patients with other conditions, who happen to be conveniently to hand. However, these are often atypical of the well population.

Selection of cases can also cause difficulties. One problem is that many conditions vary in their type and nature and it is thus difficult to decide which cases should be included. For example, if you were using a case–control design to study a possible association between attempted suicide and the use of calcium-channel blockers for hypertension, do you include all attempted suicides as cases or only those where serious intent can be reasonably established—which population are you sampling?

There is also the problem of recall bias. In case–control studies you are asking people to recall events in their past. Memories are not always reliable. Moreover, cases may have a better recall of relevant past events than controls—over the years their illness may provide more easily remembered signposts, and they have a better motive for remembering: to get better! Because of these various difficulties, case–control studies often provide results which conflict with other similar case–control studies. For reliable conclusions, cohort studies are generally preferred—but of course are not always a practical alternative.

GETTING STUCK IN: EXPERIMENTAL STUDIES

We can now turn to designs where, in contrast to observational studies, the investigators actively participate in some aspect of the recruitment, treatment or care of the subjects in the study.

Clinical Trials

Clinical trials are experiments to compare two or more clinical treatments. I use the word "treatment" here, to mean any sort of clinical intervention, from kind words to new drugs. Whole books have been written on clinical trials but I can only touch upon the some of the more important aspects of this design. Let's create the following imaginary scenario. A new drug for treating hypertension has been developed, and you have been asked to investigate its efficacy compared to the existing drug of choice, using a suitable study.

To start with, you decide that systolic blood pressure (SBP) will be your output measure. Then you need to select a sample of individuals with hypertension, and find a method of allocating them to one or other of two groups, so that the composition of the groups is as similar as possible. The groups need to be similar not only on the obvious variables, such as sex and age, but also in terms of other variables whose existence you know about but can't easily measure (like the emotional state of mind, aspects of their lifestyles, genetic differences, and so on), and similar in terms of other variables whose existence you are not even aware of.

This of course is an attempt to overcome the confounding problem. If the groups are identical in every respect (except one group got the new drug, the other the existing drug), then any reduction in blood pressure is highly likely to be due to the drug rather than to the fact that the subjects in one group are slightly older, or contained more subjects who live alone, for instance (although chance could also play a part, of course). So how do you achieve similarity in the two groups?

One group will be given the new drug, making this the *treatment group*, the other group the existing drug, making this the *control group*. A control group is imperative. If you have only one group, whose SBP you first measure, then give them the drug, then re-measure, you cannot conclude that an observed decrease in SBP is caused necessarily by the drug. Being in a calm, quiet clinical setting might reduce the SBP of all the subjects.

Randomisation

The solution to getting two groups as similar as possible is to allocate subjects using some random system, by tossing a coin maybe: heads they go to the treatment group, tails to the control group. This method has the virtue of taking the allocation out of the hands of the researcher, who might unconsciously introduce *selection bias* in the allocation, for example by choosing the least well patients for the treatment group. If the randomisation is successful, and the original sample is large enough, then the two groups should differ only by chance. This design is thus called the *randomised controlled trial* (RCT).

Coin tossing is a little impractical of course, and instead a *table of random numbers* (there's one in the Appendix) is used for the allocation process. Let's see how we might use this method to randomly allocate 15 patients. You decide to allocate a patient to the treatment group (T) if the random number is even, say, and to the control group (C) if odd. You then need to determine a starting point in the random number table, maybe by sticking a pin in the table and identifying a start number. Suppose you get the bottom row of the fourth column, where the numbers are 3 4 3 8 6. You can then go across the same row or up the column. Suppose you go up the column. The next numbers are 5 4 8 0 6 and 7 9 2 6 5. Together this give the numbers 3 4 3 8 6 5 4 8 0 6 7 9 2 6 5—which is odd, even, odd, even, even, etc. So you allocate the 15 patients as C T C T T C T T T T C C T T C—which gives you nine treatment group subjects and six control group subjects. This is a problem because you want your groups to be the same size. You can fix this by using *block randomisation*.

Block Randomisation

Here's how it works. You decide on a block size, let's say blocks of four, and write down all four-valued combinations of C and T containing *equal* numbers of Cs and Ts. Since there are six such combinations, you will have six blocks, as follows:

Block 1, CCTT;   Block 2, CTCT;   Block 3, CTTC;
Block 4, TCTC;   Block 5, TCCT;   Block 6, TTCC.

With the same random numbers as before, the first number is 3, so the first four subjects are allocated according to block 3, i.e. CTTC. The next number is 4, so the next four subjects are allocated as block 4, i.e. TCTC; and so on. Obviously random numbers greater than 6 are ignored. You carry on with this procedure until all of the subjects have been allocated to one or other of the two groups which will now be of the same size. There is more to block randomisation than this brief introduction, but space restrictions prevent me from any more detailed discussion.

Blinding

If at all possible, you don't want the patients to know whether they are in the treatment group or the control group. You can achieve this by, for example, giving them identical looking tablets. This "blinding" of the patients to their treatment is not always possible. For example, you might be testing out a new walking frame for elderly infirm patients—it will be difficult to disguise this from the older existing frame with which they are all familiar, without them noticing!

A further desirable precaution is also to blind the investigator to the allocation process. If the investigator doesn't know which subjects are receiving the drug and which the placebo, treatment of the subjects will remain impartial and even-handed. Human nature being what it is, there may be an unconscious inclination to treat a patient who is known to be in the treatment group differently from one in the control group. This effect is known as *treatment bias*, and can be avoided by blinding the investigator. We can do this by entrusting a disinterested third party to obtain the random numbers and decide on the allocation rules. Only this person will know which group any given subject is in and will not reveal this until the treatment is complete and the results collected, and analysed.

When both subject and investigator are blinded we refer to the design as a *double-blind randomised controlled trial*—the gold standard among experimental designs. Without blinding, the trial is referred to as being *open*. Compared to other designs, the RCT gives the most robust and dependable results.

The design described above in which two groups receive identical treatment (except for the difference in drugs) throughout the period of the trial is known as a *parallel* design, shown schematically in Figure 6.1.

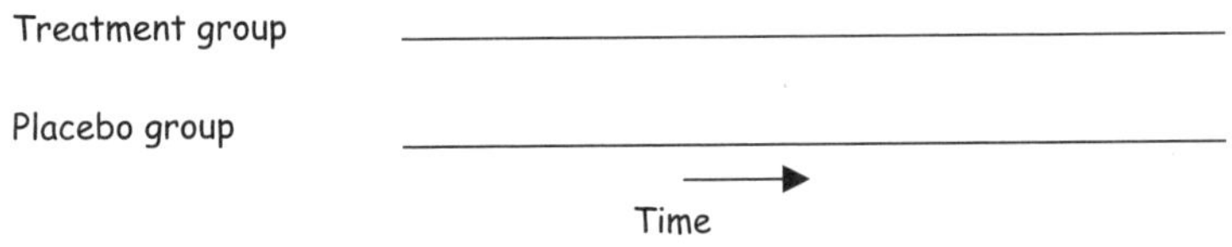

Treatment group   ——————————————————

Placebo group   ——————————————————
                              ——————▶
                          Time

Figure 6.1: Schematic of a parallel randomised controlled trial

One variant of the parallel design is to *stratify* the sample before the randomisation process, to ensure adequate representation of particular individuals in both groups, for example ethnic minority subjects.

The Cross-over Randomised Controlled Trial

A variation on the parallel design is the *cross-over* design, shown schematically in Figure 6.2. In this design one group gets drug A, say, and the second group drug B (or placebo), for some fixed period of time. Then, after a washout period to prevent drug-effect carry-over, the groups are reversed. The group which got drug A now gets drug B, and vice versa, and for the same period of time. Which group gets which treatment first is decided by randomisation.

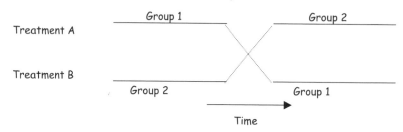

Figure 6.2:   Schematic of a cross-overall randomised controlled trial (RCT)

The advantage of this method is that each subject gets both treatments, and thus acts as his or her own control, an almost perfect match—the control subject is the same person! (Only "almost", because a subject may undergo changes between the first period and the second.) As a consequence of the matched-pair feature, this design requires smaller samples.

Needless to say, there are a number of problems with this approach. For example, it doesn't work well if the drug or treatment to be investigated requires a long time to become effective; so for practical reasons cross-over trials are generally of relatively short duration (one reason is to avoid excessive dropout). Also, despite a washout interval, there may still be a drug carry-over effect (although this can be measured). If carry-over is detected, the second half of the trial has to be abandoned. The cross-over design is also inappropriate for conditions which can be cured—most of the subjects in the active drug half might be cured by the end of the first period! In addition, the design is now experiencing ethical disapproval, although it remains popular because of its cheapness, smaller sample sizes, and quick delivery of results.

An Example from Practice

The following extract describes the design of a randomised cross-over trial of regular versus as-needed salbutamol in asthma control.

> If inclusion criteria were met at the first clinic visit, patients were enrolled in a four-week randomised crossover assessment of regular vs. as-needed salbutamol. Patients took either 2 puffs (200 pg) metered dose salbutamol from a coded inhaler or matching placebo four times

daily for two weeks. On return to the clinic, diary cards were reviewed and patients assigned to receive the crossover treatment for two weeks. During both treatment arms patients carried a salbutamol inhaler for relief of episodic asthma symptoms. Thus, the placebo treatment arm constituted as-needed salbutamol.

Patients were instructed to record their peak expiratory flow rate (PEFR) twice daily: in the early morning and late at night before inhaler use. Patients also recorded in a diary the number of daytime and night-time asthma episodes suffered and the number of as-needed salbutamol puffs used for symptom relief.

Data from the last 8 days of each treatment period were analysed; the first 6 acted as an active run-in or washout period. Two investigators, blinded to the treatment assignment, examined these comparisons for each patient and categorised each patient as showing no difference in asthma control between treatment periods, greater control during the first treatment period, greater control during the second treatment period, or differences between treatment periods that did not indicate control to be clearly better during either.

Selection of Subjects

Just a brief word about selecting subjects for the RCT. Essentially you want a sample of subjects (and they will usually be patients of some sort) who represent a cohesive and clearly defined population. Thus you might want to exclude subjects who, although they have the condition of interest, have a complicated form of it, or simultaneously have other significant illnesses or conditions, or are taking drugs for another condition—indeed anything which you feel makes them untypical of the population you have in mind.

An Example from Practice

The following extract is from a randomised controlled trial to compare the efficacy of having midwives solely manage the care of pregnant Glasgow women, with the more usual arrangements of care being shared between midwife, hospital doctors, and GPs. Outcomes were the number of interventions and complications, maternal and fetal outcomes, and maternal satisfaction with the care received. The first paragraph details the selection criteria, the second and third paragraphs describe the random allocation and the blinding processes.

> The study was carried out at Glasgow Royal Maternity Hospital, a major urban teaching hospital with around 5000 deliveries per year, serving a largely disadvantaged community. Between 11 January 1993 and 25 February 1994, all women booking for care at routine hospital-based consultant clinics were screened for eligibility; the criteria were residence within the hospital's catchment area, booking for antenatal care within 16 completed weeks of pregnancy, and absence of medical or obstetric complications (based on criteria developed by members of the clinical midwifery management team in consultation with obstetricians . . .).

> The women were randomly assigned equally between the two types of care without stratification. A restricted randomisation scheme (random permutated blocks of ten) by random number tables was prepared for each clinic by a clerical officer who was not involved in determining eligibility, administering care, or assessing outcome. The research team telephoned a clerical officer in a separate office for care allocation for each woman.

> Women in the control group had no identifying mark on their records, and clinical staff were unaware whether a particular woman was in the control group or was not in the study. We

decided not to identify control women . . . because of concern that the identification of the control group would prompt clinical staff to treat these women differently . . . .

Intention to Treat

One problem which often arises in a randomised controlled trial, after the randomisation process has taken place, is the loss of subjects, principally through dropout (moving away, refusing further treatment, dying from unrelated causes, etc.), and withdrawal for clinical reasons. Unfortunately such losses may adversely affect the balance of the two groups achieved through randomisation. In these circumstances it is good practice to analyse the data as if the lost subjects were still in the study, as you originally intended—even if not all their measurements are complete. This is known as *intention-to-treat* analysis.

Exercise 6.1
What is the fundamental difference between observational and experimental studies?

Exercise 6.2
(a) What advantages does a case–control study have over a cohort study? (b) What are the principal shortcomings of a case–control study?

Exercise 6.3
Explain how the possibility of treatment bias is overcome in the design of a randomised controlled trial.

Exercise 6.4
Using block randomisation, with blocks of four, and a random number table, allocate 40 subjects into two groups, each with 20 individuals.

Exercise 6.5
The following paragraphs contain the stated objective or hypothesis (the wording might have been changed slightly in some cases) in each of a number of recently published clinical research papers. In each case: (i) suggest a suitable outcome variable; (ii) suggest an appropriate study design or designs (there's usually more than one way to skin a cat), which would enable the investigators to achieve their stated objective(s); (iii) identify possible confounders (if appropriate); (iv) comment on the appropriateness of the designs and methods actually chosen by the researchers.

(a) To determine whether a child's tendency to atopic diseases (asthma, hay fever, excema, etc.) is associated with the number of siblings.
(b) To compare two drugs, ciprofoloxacin (CF) and pivmecillinam (PM), for the treatment of childhood shigellosis (dysentery).
(c) To study the effect of maternal chronic hypertension on the risk of small-for-gestational-age birthweight.
(d) To evaluate a possible association between maternal smoking and the birth of a Down's syndrome child.
(e) To compare, in terms of clinical efficacy and patient satisfaction, midwife-managed care of pregnant women, with conventional shared care (care shared between midwives, hospital doctors, and GPs).

(f) To compare a community-based service (patients living and treated at home) with a hospital-based service (patients admitted to and treated in hospital), for patients with acute psychiatric illness, with reference to psychiatric outcomes, the burden on relatives, and relatives' satisfaction with the service.

(g) To compare regular with as-needed inhaled salbutamol in asthma control.

(h) To evaluate the impact of counselling on: client symptomatology, self-esteem, and quality of life; drug prescribing; referrals to other mental health professionals; and client and GP satisfaction.

IV

FROM LITTLE TO LARGE: STATISTICAL INFERENCE

7

FROM SAMPLES TO POPULATIONS: MAKING INFERENCES

Learning objectives

When you have finished this chapter you should be able to:

- *Explain what a sample is, and the difference between study and target populations*
- *Show that you understand the difference, and the connection, between a population parameter and a sample statistic*
- *Explain what statistical inference is*
- *Explain what an estimate is and why this is unlikely to be exactly the same as the population parameter being estimated*

I was in the supermarket last week, trying to decide between buying red grapes or green grapes, and I did what I always do, I tried one grape from each bunch, and chose the grapes whose taste I preferred. In so doing, I was making a leap of faith, assuming that all of the other grapes in the bunch would have a similar quality to the one grape I had tasted. When you make this sort of generalisation you are *inferring*. Inferring simply means guessing or concluding or assuming something, on the basis of some information or evidence. In this example, I was inferring something about the quality of the whole bunch of grapes, on the evidence provided by one grape from the bunch.

In statistics we do much the same thing all the time, and we call it *statistical inference*, although of course the setting is different! In fact, statistical inference is the rationale for most of the statistical procedures discussed in this book. For example, suppose you want to determine the percentage of women in the UK with genital chlamydia. You obviously can't examine every woman in the country, there are far too many of them, you don't have all their names and addresses, and some would certainly decline an examination anyway. So you need to find a group of women, a *sample*, which you think is typical or representative of the *population* of all UK women.

I am not using the word "population" in its geographical sense here (i.e. to mean everybody living in a country or region). In statistics, a population is whatever you define it to be. If you were interested only in all single women aged under 30 in the UK, *this* would be your population; if only in all single women attending your well-women clinic in Leeds, *this* would be your population.[1] Statisticians refer to the *target population*, meaning the greater, inaccessible population (all women in the UK, for example), and the *study population*, meaning that group of individuals who are actually available and from whom the sample could actually be taken. This might be all women attending your well-women clinics.

Let's now assume that in your sample of women you find that 2.5% have genital chlamydia, so your informed guess or *estimate* is that 2.5% of all UK women have genital chlamydia. You have inferred something about a population on the basis of some sample evidence. This is statistical inference. I have used the word "estimate" here deliberately, because the value you get from your sample (from *any* sample) is never going to be exactly the same as the population value, because no sample is completely identical with the population it is taken from.[2] You have to accept that the percentage with genital chlamydia in the population is probably around 2.5%, *give or take a bit*. The size of the "bit" depends on how similar your sample is to its population—ultimately to chance. I'll have a lot more to say on this later in the book.

This is a problem that you should always be aware of in both your own work and that of others. A sample can be assumed to be representative only of the population which was available to be sampled. The degree to which this population is typical of the target population is always questionable. I am going to deal with the question of obtaining representative samples in the next chapter.

Now, the meaning of a few terms. The feature or characteristic of a population whose value you want to determine is known as a *population parameter*. The mean of some variable in a population, or the median, or the standard deviation, are all population parameters. Their values *define* that population. In the genital chlamydia example, the population parameter you want to estimate is the *percentage* with genital chlamydia.

The value that you get from your sample, in this case the *sample percentage* with genital chlamydia (on which you are going to base your estimate of the population value), is called the *sample statistic*. This is why we are so interested in the summary descriptive measures (such as the sample mean, the sample median, and so on) described in Chapter 6. These are the sample statistics on which you will base your inferences. In other words, you can use the sample mean, for example, to estimate the population mean, the sample median to estimate the population median, and so on.

To sum up:

> Statistical inference is the process of using a value obtained from the sample, known as the sample statistic, to estimate the value of the corresponding population parameter.

---

[1] Most clinical investigations involve populations of people (often patients) as the subjects of any study, but the subjects could be cervical smears (how many are misclassified), or crash trolleys (what percentage are completely equipped), and so on.
[2] An estimate is just a fancy word for an informed guess.

The idea of using a sample statistic to estimate a population parameter is shown schematically in Figure 7.1, using the genital chlamydia question as an example.

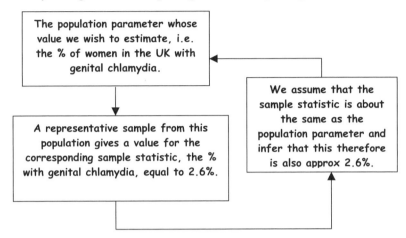

Figure 7.1:   Schematic of the process of statistical inference

Actually, estimation is not the only way of making inferences about population parameter values. An alternative approach is to first make an (informed) assumption about the value of some population parameter, and then use the appropriate sample statistic to see whether its value supports your assumption. This approach is called *hypothesis testing*. In Chapters 9 to 11, I discuss some common estimation procedures, and in Chapters 12 to 14 the alternative hypothesis test approach. Before any of this, however, I need to introduce the idea of probability and some other important stuff. This is what I will do in the following chapter.

Exercise 7.1
Explain the meaning of, and the difference between, a population parameter and a sample statistic. (b) Why is a sample, however well chosen, never going to be *exactly* representative of the sampled population? (c) What is the difference between a target population and a study population?

8

PROBABILITY, RISK, AND ODDS

Learning objectives

When you have finished this chapter you should be able to:

- *Define probability, explain what an event is, and calculate simple probabilities*
- *Explain the proportional frequency approach to calculating probability*
- *Explain how probability can be used with the area properties of the Normal distribution, and calculate probability in this context*
- *Define and explain the idea of risk and its relationship with probability*
- *Calculate the risk of some outcome from a contingency table, and interpret the result*
- *Define and explain the idea of odds*
- *Calculate odds from a case–control 2 × 2 table, and interpret the result*
- *State the equation linking probability and odds, and be able to calculate one, given the other*
- *Explain what the risk ratio of some outcome is, calculate a risk ratio, and interpret the result*
- *Explain what the odds ratio for some outcome is, calculate an odds ratio, and interpret the result*
- *Explain why it's not possible to calculate a risk ratio in a case–control study*
- *Define number needed to treat, explain its use, and calculate NNT in a simple example*

Chance Would Be a Fine Thing: the Idea of Probability

Put simply, probability is a measure of the chance of getting some particular outcome, when you perform some *experiment*. By "experiment", I mean any process whose outcome is uncertain. For example, rolling a dice (with six possible outcomes, 1 to 6), taking a biopsy (two possible outcomes, benign or malignant), determining an Apgar score for an infant (11 possible outcomes, from 0 to 10), and so on.

If some particular outcome is *certain* to happen, we say it has a probability of 1; if it is *impossible*, we say it has a probability of 0. Throwing a 7 with a normal dice is impossible, so this outcome has a probability of 0. Throwing a number between 1 and 6 is certain, so has a probability of 1. Thus the probability of any outcome varies from 0 to 1. Incidentally, the word "risk" is synonymous with "probability".

Statisticians tend to use the word *event* rather than outcome, and then define an event as some particular outcome, or *combination* of outcomes. For example, the event "rolling an even number when throwing a dice" is a combination of the outcomes, rolling a 2 or rolling a 4 or rolling a 6.

The probability, p, of an event X, written as $p(X)$, can vary from 0 to 1. Mathematically this can be expressed as

$0 \le p(X) \le 1.$

$$0 \le p(x) \le 1$$

CALCULATING PROBABILITY

You can calculate the probability of a particular event using the following expression:

Probability of an event = The number of outcomes which favour that event divided by the *total* number of possible outcomes.

Take a simple example. Suppose you are playing Snakes and Ladders, and it's your turn to roll the dice. Throwing an even number will take you up a ladder, but throwing an odd number will slide you down a snake. What is the probability of the event "you will go up a ladder"? There are three favourable outcomes, 2, 4 or 6, out of the six possible outcomes, 1, 2, 3, 4, 5 or 6. If you divide the former number by the latter, the probability you want is:

Probability of getting 2, 4 or 6, and hence going up a ladder = 3/6 = 0.5.

The fact that this probability is half way between 0 and 1 implies that getting an even number is just as likely as getting an odd number—you're just as likely to go up a ladder as down a snake. Such is life.

The above method for determining probability works well with experiments where all of the outcomes have the same probability, such as rolling dice, tossing a coin, etc. In the real world you will often have to use what is called the *proportional frequency* approach, which uses existing frequency data as the basis for probability calculations. As an example, refer back to Figure 2.1, the frequency table showing the distribution of Apgar scores in 30 infants. I have reproduced this as Table 8.1, and added an extra column showing the *proportional* frequency— category frequency divided by total frequency. Notice that the proportional frequencies sum to 1.

Now ask the question, "What is the probability that if you chose one of these 30 infants at random it will have an Apgar score of 9?" The answer is the proportional frequency for the "Apgar score = 9" category, i.e. 3/30 or 0.1000. In other words, we can interpret proportions as equivalent to probabilities. Now a slightly harder question: what is the probability that an infant will have an Apgar score

Table 8.1   Proportional frequencies for the Apgar scores of 30 infants

APGAR SCORE	NUMBER OF INFANTS (frequency)	PROPORTIONAL FREQUENCY
4	2	0.0667
5	3	0.1000
6	6	0.2000
7	7	0.2333
8	9	0.3000
9	3	0.1000

less than 7? Now, the event of interest is a score of 6 or 5 or 4 or 3 or 2 or 1 or 0. But each of these outcomes is *mutually exclusive*, because if a particular infant has an Apgar score of 6 then that infant can't have any of the other Apgar scores.

When outcomes are mutually exclusive like this, then the probability of the event involved is equal to the *sum* of the individual probabilities. In this case the sum of the individual probabilities, or proportional frequencies (because they're the same thing here), for the Apgar scores from 0 up to 6 is:

  0.000 + 0.0000 + 0.000 + 0.0000 + 0.0667 + 0.1000 + 0.2000 = 0.3667

So the probability of an infant having an Apgar score less than 7 is just over a third, or one infant in three. Notice that the probability of some event *not* happening is (1 minus the probability that it will happen). For example, the probability of an infant having an Apgar score of 7 *or more* is (1 − 0.3667) = 0.6333.

Exercise 8.1
Figure 1.2 shows the basic characteristics of the two groups of women receiving a breast lump diagnosis in the stress and breast cancer study. What is the probability that a woman chosen at random: (a) will have had her breast lump diagnosed as (i) benign, (ii) malignant? (b) will be post-menopausal? (c) will have had more than one child?

Exercise 8.2
Figure 1.3 is from a study of thrombotic risk during pregnancy. What is the probability (under classification 1) that a subject chosen at random will be aged (a) less than 30, (b) more than 29?

PROBABILITY AND THE NORMAL DISTRIBUTION

Look again at the area properties of the Normal distribution in Figure 5.5. If data is Normally distributed then 95% of the values will lie no further than two standard deviations from the mean. In probability terms, there is an equivalent probability of 0.95 that a single value chosen at random from the set of values will lie no further than two standard deviations from the mean. In the case of the Normally distributed birthweight data, this means that there is a probability of 0.95 that the birthweight of one of these infants chosen at random will be between 2513g and 4775g.

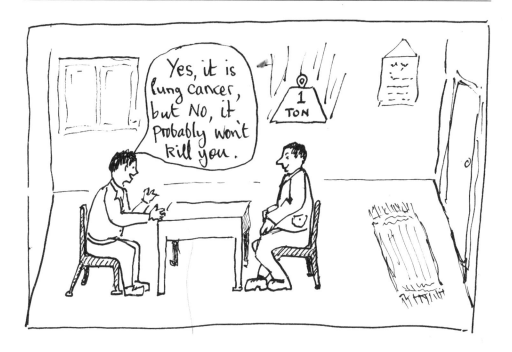

Exercise 8.3

Using the information on cord platelet count in Figure 4.5, determine the probability that one infant chosen at random from this sample will have a cord platelet count: (a) between $101 \times 10^9/L$ and $515 \times 10^9/L$; (b) less than $239 \times 10^9/L$.

RISK

As I mentioned earlier, a *risk* is the same as a probability, but the former word tends to be favoured in the clinical arena. So the definition of probability, given earlier in a box, applies equally here to risk:

> Risk of an event = Number of favourable outcomes divided by the total number of outcomes.

Since it's a probability, risk can vary between 0 and 1. As an example, and also to re-visit the contingency table, look again at the table in Table 6.1 from the cohort study of coronary heart disease (CHD) in adult life, and weighing 18lb or less at one year, which we are treating as a risk factor.

The risk (or probability) that those adults who as infants weighed 18lb or less at one year will have CHD is equal to the number who weighed 18lb or less at one year and had CHD, divided by the total number who weighed 18lb or less, which equals 4/15 = 0.2667. Similarly, the risk (or probability) for those who weighed more than 18lb at one year will have CHD equals the number who weighed more than 18lb at one year and had CHD, divided by the total number who weighed more than 18lb = 38/275 = 0.1382, which is only half the risk of those weighing 18lb or less.

The risk for a single group, as it is described above, is also known as the *absolute risk*, mainly to distinguish it from *relative risk*—that is, the risk for one group *compared* to the risk for some other group (I'll deal with this shortly).

Exercise 8.4

Table 8.2 is from a cohort study into the influence of sex, age, body mass index (BMI) and smoking, on alcohol intake and mortality, in Danish men and women aged between 30 and 79 years. The table shows the distribution of alcohol intake and deaths by sex and level of alcohol intake. Use the information in the table to construct an appropriate contingency table, and calculate for (a) men and (b) women the absolute risk of death among those subjects who consume (i) less than 1 beverage a week, (ii) more than 69 beverages a week. Interpret your results.

Table 8.2 Distribution of alcohol intake and deaths by sex and level of alcohol intake from a cohort study into the influence of sex, age, body mass index, and smoking on alcohol intake and mortality

ALCOHOL INTAKE (beverages a week)*	MEN		WOMEN	
	No. of subjects	No. (%) of deaths	No. of subjects	No. (%) of deaths
<1	625	195 (31.2)	2472	394 (15.9)
1–6	1183	252 (21.3)	3079	283 (9.2)
7–13	1825	383 (21.0)	1019	96 (9.4)
14–27	1234	285 (23.1)	543	46 (8.5)
28–41	585	118 (20.2)	72	6 (8.3)
42–69	388	99 (25.5)	29	5 (17.2)
>69	211	66 (31.3)	20	1 (5.0)
Total	6051	1398 (23.1)	7234	831 (11.5)

*One beverage contains 9–13g alcohol.

ODDS

As you saw above, the probability (or risk) of an event is the number of favourable outcome divided by the *total* number of outcomes, but the *odds* for an event is:

> Odds for an event = The number of outcomes favourable to the event divided by the number of outcomes not favourable to the event.

Notice that the value for odds can vary from 0 to infinity, with the following implications:

- When the odds for an event are less than 1, the odds are unfavourable; the event is less likely to happen than it is to happen.

- When the odds equal 1, the event is as likely to happen as not.
- When the odds are greater than 1, the odds are favourable; the event is more likely to happen than not.

If you go back to the dice rolling game, the *odds* in favour of the event "an even number" is the number of outcomes favourable to the event (the number of even numbers, i.e. 2, 4, 6), divided by the number of outcomes not favourable to the event (the number of *not* even numbers, i.e. 1, 3, 5), which is 3/3 = 1/1. So the odds for this event are "evens"—the odds of getting an even number are the same as the odds of getting an odd number. Nearly all the odds in health statistics are expressed as "something" to 1. We call this value of 1 the *reference value*.

As a further example, using the Apgar scores in Figure 2.1, the odds in favour of an infant having an Apgar score of less than 7 is the number of values *less* than 7, divided by the number of values *not* less than 7, or 11/19 = 0.58/1, or just 0.58.

We can also calculate odds from a table such as that for the exercise and stroke case–control study in Table 6.2. Among those patients who'd had a stroke, 55 had exercised (been exposed to the risk), and 70 had not, so the odds that those with a stroke had exercised is 55/70 = 0.7857. Among those patients who hadn't had a stroke, 130 had exercised and 68 had not, so the odds that they had exercised is 130/68 = 1.9118. In other words, among those who had had a stroke, the odds that they had exercised was only about half the odds (0.7857/1.9118) of those who hadn't had a stroke. Exercise when young seems to confer protection against a stroke.

Exercise 8.5

Table 8.3 is from a case–control study into maternal smoking during pregnancy and Down's syndrome, and shows the basic characteristics of mothers giving birth to babies with Down's syndrome (cases), and without Down's syndrome (controls). Use the information in the table to construct an appropriate 2 × 2 table, for women (a) aged under 35, and (b) aged 35 and over. Hence calculate the odds among mothers giving birth to (i) a Down's syndrome baby, and (ii) a healthy baby, that they had smoked during pregnancy. What do you conclude?

Why You Can't Calculate Risk in a Case–Control Study

For most people the *risk* of an event, being akin to probability, makes more sense and is easier to interpret than the odds for that same event, which is a bit of a fuzzy concept. That being so, maybe it would be more helpful to express the stroke/exercise result as a risk rather than as odds. Unfortunately we can't, and here's why.

To calculate the risk that those with a stroke had exercised, you need to know two things, the total number who'd had a stroke, and the number of these who had been exposed to the risk (of exercise). You then divide the latter by the former. In a cohort study you would select the groups on this basis, whether they had been exposed to the risk (of exercising) or not. So one group would contain individuals exposed to the risk and the other those not exposed.

Table 8.3 Basic characteristics of mothers in a case–control study of maternal smoking and Down's syndrome

	CASES (n = 775)		CONTROLS (n = 7750)	
	No.	%	No.	%
Age (years)				
<20	50	6.5	801	10.3
20–24	143	18.5	2092	27.0
25–29	163	21.0	2431	31.4
30–34	205	26.5	1664	21.5
≥35	214	27.6	762	9.8
Race				
White	629	81.2	6322	81.6
Hispanic	68	8.8	450	5.8
Black	22	2.8	289	3.7
American Indian	14	1.8	171	2.2
Other	31	4.0	395	5.1
Unknown	11	1.4	123	1.6
Marital status				
Married	614	79.2	6016	77.6
Unmarried	161	20.8	1717	22.2
Unknown			17	0.2
Smoking during pregnancy				
Age <35 years				
Yes	112	20.0	1411	20.2
No	421	75.0	5214	74.6
Unknown	28	5.0	363	5.2
Age ≥35 years				
Yes	15	7.0	108	14.2
No	186	86.9	611	80.2
Unknown	13	6.1	43	5.6
Parity (Age <35 years)				
0	214	38.1	2933	42.0
1	186	33.2	2261	32.4
2	88	15.7	1053	15.1
≥3	67	11.9	573	8.2
Unknown	6	1.1	168	2.4

But in a case–control study you don't select on the basis of whether people have been exposed to the risk or not, but on the basis of whether they have some condition (a stroke) or not. So you have one group composed of individuals who have the condition and one group who don't, but *both* groups will contain individuals who were and were not exposed to the risk (of exercising). Moreover, you can select whatever number of cases and controls you want. You could for example halve the number of cases and double the number of controls. This means the column totals, which you would otherwise need for your risk calculation, are meaningless.

THE LINK BETWEEN PROBABILITY AND ODDS

If you study the definitions of probability (risk) and odds on pages 85 and 88, you won't be surprised that you can derive one from another:

Risk or probability = odds/(1 + odds)

Odds = probability/(1 − probability)

Exercise 8.6

Following on from Exercise 8.5, what is the probability that a mother aged ≥35 chosen at random from (a) mothers of Down syndrome babies, (b) mothers of healthy babies, will have smoked during pregnancy?

THE RISK RATIO

In practice, risks and odds for a single group are not nearly as interesting as a *comparison* of risks and odds between two groups. For risk you can make these comparisons by dividing the risk for one group (usually the group exposed to the risk factor) by the risk for the second, non-exposed group. This gives us the *risk ratio*.[1] Let's calculate the risk ratio for the data in Table 6.1, from the cohort study of coronary heart disease (CHD) in adult life, and weighing 18lb or less at one year, using the results obtained on pages 87–88:

Among those weighing ≤18lb at one year, risk of CHD = 0.2667

Among those weighing >18lb at one year, risk of CHD = 0.1382.

So the risk *ratio* for CHD among those weighing 18lb or less at one year compared to those weighing more than 18lb = 0.2667/0.1382 = 1.9298. We interpret this as follows: adults who weighed 18lb or less at one year old have nearly twice the risk of CHD as those who weighed more than 18lb.

We can generalise the risk ratio calculation with the help of the contingency table in Table 8.4, where the cell values are represented as a, b, c and d. Among those exposed to the risk factor, the risk of disease is $a/(a + c)$. Among those not exposed, the risk of disease is $b/(b + d)$. Therefore:

$$\text{Risk ratio} = \frac{\dfrac{a}{(a + c)}}{\dfrac{b}{(b + d)}} = \frac{a(b + d)}{b(a + c)}.$$

Table 8.4   Generalised contingency table for risk ratio calculations in a cohort study

OUTCOME: has disease	GROUP BY EXPOSED TO RISK FACTOR		
	Yes	*No*	Totals
Yes	a	b	$(a + b)$
No	c	d	$(c + d)$
Totals	$(a + c)$	$(b + d)$	

---

[1] Risk ratio is also known as *relative risk*.

Exercise 8.7

Use the results you obtained in Exercise 8.4 to calculate the risk ratio of death for those who consumed more than 69 beverages a week, compared with those who consumed less than 1 beverage per week, which we'll define as the reference group, for (a) men and (b) women. Interpret your results.

THE ODDS RATIO

With a case–control study you can similarly compare the odds that those with a disease will have been exposed to the risk factor with the odds that those who don't have the disease will have been exposed. If you divide the former by the latter you get the *odds ratio*. On page 89 you calculated the following odds for the stroke and exercise study (where we are treating exercise as the risk factor): the odds that those with a stroke had exercised are $55/70 = 0.7857$; and the odds that those without a stroke had exercised are $130/68 = 1.9118$. Dividing the former by the latter, you get the odds ratio $0.7857/1.9118 = 0.4110$.

This result suggests that those with a stroke are less than half as likely to have exercised when young as the healthy controls. It would seem that exercise is a *beneficial* "risk" factor. We can generalise the odds ratio calculation with the help of the 2×2 chart in Table 8.5, where the cell values are represented as a, b, c and d. The odds of exposure to the risk factor among those with the disease is a/c, and the odds of exposure to the risk factor among the healthy controls is b/d. Therefore:

$$\text{Odds ratio} = \frac{a/c}{b/d} = ad/bc.$$

Table 8.5   Generalised 2×2 table for odds ratio calculations in a case–control study

EXPOSED TO RISK FACTOR	GROUP BY OUTCOME (e.g. disease)	
	Cases	*Controls*
Yes	a	b
No	c	d

Exercise 8.8

Use the results from Exercise 8.5 to calculate the odds ratio for smoking among the mothers of Down's syndrome babies compared to mothers of healthy babies, for (a) mothers aged under 35, (b) mothers aged 35 and over. Interpret your results.

Remember that the risk and odds ratios in the coronary heart disease and in the stroke examples above are *sample* risk and odds ratios. For instance, from the *sample* risk ratio of 1.93 (1.9298 to two decimal places) in the CHD/weight at one year study, you can infer that the *population* risk ratio is also *about* 1.93 plus or minus (±) a "bit". But how big is this "bit", how precise is your estimate? That is a question I'll address in Chapter 11.

Finally, I mentioned earlier that most people are happier with the concept of "risk" than with "odds", but that you can't calculate risk in a case–control study. However, there is a happy ending. The odds ratio in a case–control study is a reasonably good estimator of the equivalent risk ratio, so although you can't actually calculate the risk ratio in a case–control study, you can at least approximate its value with the corresponding odds ratio. This means you can provide a risk measure which is generally more readily understood.

NUMBERS NEEDED TO TREAT (NNT)

This seems as good a time as any to discuss a measure of the effectiveness of a clinical procedure which is related to risk, more precisely to absolute risk—this is the *numbers needed to treat*, or NNT. It is the number of patients who would need to be treated with the active procedure rather than a placebo (or alternative procedure) in order to reduce by one the number of patients experiencing the condition. To explain NNT let's go back to the example for weighing 18lb or less at one year as a risk factor for coronary heart disease (CHD). The absolute risk of CHD among those weighing 18lb or less was 0.2667. The absolute risk of CHD for those weighing more than 18lb was 0.1382. So the *absolute risk reduction* (ARR) is the difference in these two absolute risks. It's the reduction in risk gained by weighing more than 18lb at one year rather than weighing 18lb or less. In this case:

ARR = 0.2667 − 0.1382 = 0.1285.

Now NNT is defined as follows:

NNT = 1/ARR;

so:

NNT = 1/0.1285 = 7.78.

This means that if you had some treatment (infant-care advice for vulnerable parents, for example), which would cause infants who would otherwise have weighed less than 18lb at one year to weigh 18lb or more, then you would need to "treat" eight infants (or their parents) to ensure that one patient did not have coronary heart disease.[2] NNT is often used to give a familiar and practical meaning to outcomes from clinical trials, and systematic reviews,[3] where measures of risk and risk ratios may be difficult to translate into the potential benefit to patients.

An Example from Practice

Table 8.6 is from the follow-up (cohort) study into the effectiveness of carotid endarterectomy in ipsilateral stroke prevention referred to in Figure 3.2. The table shows that, for any stroke, the (absolute) risk if treated medically is 0.110 (11.0%), and if treated

---

[2] The number must always be rounded up.
[3] Systematic review is the systematic collection of all the results from as many similarly-designed studies as possible dealing with the same clinical problem. I don't have the space in this book to discuss this procedure.

surgically is 0.051 (5.1%). The reduction in absolute risk, ARR, is thus $0.110 - 0.051 = 0.059$ (5.9%). So NNT = $1/0.059 = 16.95$ or 17, at five years. In other words, 17 patients would have to be treated with carotid endarterectomy to prevent one patient from having a stroke who, without the treatment, would otherwise have done so within five years.

Table 8.6   Example of percentage numbers needed to treat (NNT) at five years and two years from a follow-up (cohort) study into the effectiveness of carotid endarterectomy in stroke prevention

CAUSE	MEDICALLY TREATED GROUP	SURGICALLY TREATED GROUP	REDUCTION IN RISK	ABSOLUTE DIFFERENCE IN RISK	NO NEED TO TREAT*	
					At 5 years	At 2 years
Any stroke†	11.0	5.1	54	5.9	17	67
Large-artery stroke‡	6.6	3.1	54	3.5	29	111

*The number needed to treat is calculated as the reciprocal of the difference in risk. At two years, the number needed to treat is based on estimated differences in risk of 1.5% for stroke of any cause and 0.9% for large-artery stroke.
†The risk of stroke from any cause in the medical and surgical groups in the Asymptomatic Carotid Atherosclerosis Study is shown.
‡The estimates of the risk of large-artery stroke were based on the observations that for subjects in the NASCET with 60 to 99% stenosis, the ratio of the risk of large-artery stroke to the risk of stroke from any cause in the territory of a symptomatic artery was similar in the medically and surgically treated subjects, and the risk of large-artery stroke was approximately 60% of the risk of stroke from any cause in the territory of an asymptomatic artery (i.e. 6.6% = 60% of 11.0%, and 3.1% = 60% of 5.1%).

Exercise 8.9

In a cohort study of a possible connection between dental disease and coronary heart disease (CHD), subjects were tracked for 14 years. Of 3542 subjects with no dental disease, 92 died from CHD, while of 1786 subjects with periodontitis, 151 died from CHD. How many people must be successfully treated for periodontitis to prevent one person dying from CHD?

V

THE INFORMED GUESS: CONFIDENCE INTERVAL ESTIMATION

9

ESTIMATING THE VALUE OF A *SINGLE* POPULATION PARAMETER

Learning objectives

When you have finished this chapter you should be able to:

- Describe the sampling distribution of the sample mean, and the characteristics of its distribution
- Explain what the standard error of the sample mean is, and calculate its value
- Explain how you can use the probability properties of the Normal distribution to measure the preciseness of the sample mean as an estimator of the population mean, and hence derive an expression for the confidence interval of the population mean
- Calculate and interpret a 95% confidence interval for the population mean
- Calculate and interpret a 95% confidence interval for the population proportion
- Explain and interpret a 95% confidence interval for the population median

The Informed Guess

You saw in Chapter 5 that you can use a sample statistic, such as the sample mean birthweight of the 30 infants in Table 2.1, to make an informed guess, or *estimate*, of the value of the corresponding population parameter, such as the mean birthweight of *all* infants of whom this sample is representative. The sample mean birthweight was 3644.4g, so you can estimate the population mean birthweight also to be *about* 3644g, plus or minus some (hopefully) small random or *sampling error*, caused by the fact that the sample won't represent the population exactly. Incidentally, the value of the sample mean of 3644.4g is known as the *point estimate* of the population mean. It's the *single best guess* you could make as to the value of the population mean (but of course you know that it would be a miracle if your population mean was *exactly* equal to 3644.4g).

The natural question is, how small is this plus or minus bit? Can it be quantified? Can we establish how precise our sample mean birthweight is as an estimate of population mean birthweight? Put another way, how close to the population mean can you expect any given sample mean to be? To answer these questions you will need to use what is known as the *standard error*. The easiest way to explain standard error is with the confidence interval estimator of a single population mean.

ESTIMATING A CONFIDENCE INTERVAL FOR THE MEAN OF A SINGLE POPULATION

The Standard Error of the Mean

Our sample of 30 infants produced a sample mean birthweight of 3644.4g. You could take a second, different, sample of 30, which would produce another value for the sample mean. And a third sample, and a fourth, and so on. In fact from any realistic population you could (in theory) take a huge number of different same-size samples, each of which would produce a different sample mean. If you were now to arrange all of these sample means into a frequency curve, you would find that it was Normal, and centred around the true population mean. In other words, the mean of all possible sample means is the same as the population mean. This is very reassuring: it means that *on average* the sample mean estimates the population mean exactly. But note the "on average"—a particular single sample mean may still be some distance from the true mean.

We can measure the spread of the distribution of sample means in the usual way, by calculating its standard deviation, except that in the context of a sampling distribution like this we call it the "standard error of the sampling distribution of the sample mean"—quite a mouthful, but known more familiarly as the *standard error of the mean*, and abbreviated as SE ($\bar{x}$), where the symbol $\bar{x}$ stands for the sample mean. The size of a standard error is inversely linked to n, the size of the samples, by the equation:

$$SE(\bar{x}) = s/\sqrt{n}.$$

Here s is the sample standard deviation, and n is the sample size, so it's not difficult to calculate a standard error for the single sample mean by hand (although first calculating s is tedious). Clearly the larger the sample size, the smaller the standard error—since larger samples are likely to be more representative of the population. The smaller the standard error, the narrower is the spread of all the sample mean values around the population mean, and the closer therefore to the population mean any single sample mean is likely to be. This is important because in practice you usually get to take only one sample, not many. This idea is illustrated in Figure 9.1 which shows two sampling distributions of the sample mean, one for small samples and one for large samples.

To sum up, the standard error is a measure of the preciseness of the sample mean as an estimator of the population mean. Smaller is better. If you are comparing the precision of two different sample means as estimates of a population mean, the sample mean with the smallest standard error is the more precise.

Exercise 9.1

A team of researchers used a cohort study to investigate the intake of vitamins E, C and A, and the risk of lung cancer. For vitamins E and C, they calculated the mean intake (and SE) of individuals with lung cancer (the cases) and without (non-cases), after 19 years. Vitamin E, cases: 6.03mg (0.35mg); non-cases: 6.30mg (0.05mg). Vitamin C, cases:

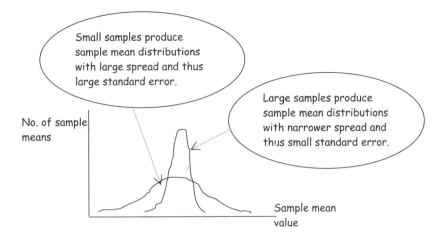

Figure 9.1: With small samples, the distribution of sample means has a wide spread, the standard error is large, and any one particular sample mean *could* be a long way from the population mean. In other words the sample mean is an imprecise estimator of the population mean. With large samples, the distribution of sample means is narrower, the standard error is smaller, and any one particular sample mean is likely to be closer to the population mean. The sample mean is a more precise estimator of the population mean

64.18mg (5.06mg); non-cases: 82.21mg (0.80mg). Comment on the likely precision of these four sample means.

Using the SE of the Mean to Calculate a Confidence Interval for a Single Population Mean

We can use the fact that the distribution of all possible sample means is Normally distributed to quantify how close to the population mean any particular sample mean is likely to be. Recall from Chapter 5 that one of the properties of any Normally distributed variable is that 95% of all values will lie in the interval (the mean ± two standard deviations). The variable here is the sample mean, and since the standard deviation is the same as the standard error, you can say that 95% of all sample means will lie in the interval (the population mean ± two standard errors). That is:

Sample mean = population mean ± 2 × standard error.

With a bit of manipulation we can rearrange this as:

Population mean = sample mean ± 2 × standard error.

To put it in words:

- We can be 95% confident that the interval, from the sample mean minus 2 × standard error, to the sample mean plus 2 × standard error, will include the population mean.
- Or in probability terms, there is a probability of 0.95 that the interval from the sample mean minus 2 × standard error, to the sample mean plus 2 × standard error, will contain the population mean.

In other words, if you pick one of all the possible sample means at random, there is a probability of 0.95, that it will lie within two standard errors of the population mean.[1] We call the distance from the sample mean minus 2SE to the sample mean plus 2SE, the *confidence interval*.

The above result means that you now quantify just how close a sample mean is likely to be to the population mean. For obvious reasons the value you get when you put some figures into this expression is known as the *95% confidence interval estimator* of the population mean. A 95% *confidence level* is most common, but 99% confidence intervals are also used. Note that the confidence interval is sometimes said to represent a *plausible range of values* for the population parameter.

An Example from Practice

In the cord-platelet count histogram in Figure 4.5, the mean cord platelet count in a sample of 4382 infants is $306 \times 10^9/L$, and the standard deviation is $69 \times 10^9/L$, so the standard error of the mean is:

$$SE(\bar{x}) = 69 \times 10^9/\sqrt{4382} = 1.042 \times 10^9/L.$$

Therefore the 95% confidence interval for the population mean cord platelet count is:

$$(306 - 2 \times 1.042 \text{ to } 306 + 2 \times 1.042)g \text{ or } (303.916 \text{ to } 308.084) \times 10^9/L.$$

This means that we can be 95% confident that the population mean cord platelet count is between $303.916 \times 10^9/L$ and $308.084 \times 10^9/L$, or alternatively that there's a probability of 0.95 that the interval from 303.916 to 308.084 will contain the population mean value. Of course there's also a 5% chance (or a 0.05 probability), that it will not! Alternatively we can say that the interval (303.916 to 308.084) $\times 10^9/L$ represents a plausible range of values for the population mean cord platelet count.

The narrower the confidence interval the more precise is the estimator. In the cord platelet example, the small width, and therefore high precision of the confidence interval is due to the large sample. By the way, it's good practice to put the confidence interval in brackets and use the "to" in the middle and not a "–" sign, since this may be confusing if the confidence interval has a negative value.

Exercise 9.2
Use the summary age measures given in Table 1.2 to calculate the standard error and 95% confidence intervals for population mean age of (a) the cases, and (b) the controls. Interpret your confidence intervals. What do you make of the fact that the two confidence intervals don't overlap?

---

[1] I have used the value 2 in all of these expressions as a convenient approximation to the exact value (which in any case will be very close to 2, when the probability is 0.95), which comes from what is known as the *t-distribution*. The t-distribution is similar to the Normal distribution, but for small sample sizes is slightly wider and flatter, and is used instead of the Normal distribution for reasons connected to inferences about the population standard deviation. Anyway, in practice you will use a computer to obtain your confidence interval result. This will use the correct value.

An Example from Practice

The results in Table 9.1 are from a randomised trial to evaluate the use of an integrated care scheme for asthma patients, in which care is shared between the GP and a specialist chest physician. The treatment group patients each received this integrated care, the control group conventional care from their GP only. The researchers were interested in the differences between the groups, if any, in a number of outcomes, shown in the figure (ignore the last column for now). The target population they have in mind is probability all asthma patients in the UK.

Table 9.1   Means and 95% confidence intervals for a number of clinical outcomes over 12 months, from a randomised trial to evaluate an integrated care scheme for asthma patients. The treatment group patients received integrated care, the control group conventional GP care

CLINICAL OUTCOME	INTEGRATED CARE (n ≥296)	CONVENTIONAL CARE (n ≥277)	RATIO OF MEANS
No. of bronchodilators prescribed	10.1 (9.2 to 11.1)	10.6 (9.7 to 11.7)	0.95 (0.83 to 1.09)
No. of inhaled steroids prescribed	6.4 (5.9 to 6.9)	6.5 (6.1 to 7.1)	0.98 (0.88 to 1.09)
No. of courses of oral steroids used	1.6 (1.4 to 1.8)	1.6 (1.4 to 1.9)	0.97 (0.79 to 1.20)
No. of general practice asthma consultations	2.7 (2.4 to 3.1)	2.5 (2.2 to 2.8)	1.11 (0.95 to 1.31)
No. of hospital admissions for asthma	0.15 (0.11 to 0.19)	0.11 (0.08 to 0.15)	1.31 (0.87 to 1.96)

Means and 95% confidence interval are estimated from Poisson regression models after controlling for initial peak flow, forced expiratory volume (as % of predicted), and duration of asthma.

You can see that in the integrated care group of 296 subjects, the *sample* mean number of bronchodilators prescribed over 12 months was 10.1, with a 95% confidence interval for the *population* mean of (9.2 to 11.1). So you can be 95% confident that the population mean number of bronchodilators prescribed for this group is somewhere between 9.2 and 11.1 . In the control group, the sample mean is 10.6 with a 95% confidence interval for the population mean (9.7 to 11.7), which can be similarly interpreted.

Exercise 9.3
Interpret and compare the sample mean number of hospital admissions, and their corresponding confidence intervals, for the two groups in Table 9.1.

ESTIMATING A CONFIDENCE INTERVAL FOR THE PROPORTION (OR PERCENTAGE) OF A SINGLE POPULATION

If you have some sample data on the smoking status of each individual in a group, it's easy enough to calculate the proportion or percentage of individuals in the sample who smoke (see Chapter 5). You can then use this sample value to calculate a confidence interval for the population proportion or percentage. As usual you will want to use a computer program to do all the work for you, but if you need to calculate it by hand, the standard error of the sample proportion is:

$$SE(p) = \sqrt{\frac{p(1-p)}{n}}$$

where p is the sample proportion and n is sample size. Incidentally, the sampling distribution of sample proportions has a binomial distribution, which is quite

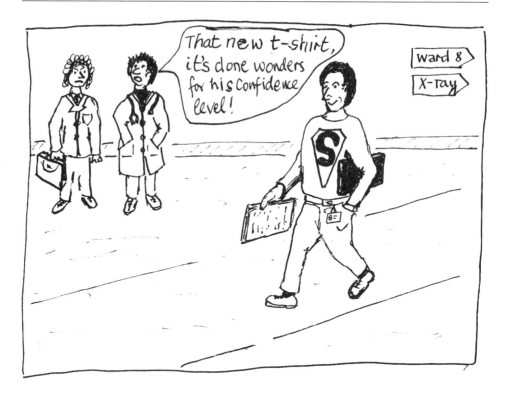

different from the Normal distribution if the sample is small, but becomes more Normal as sample size increases.

The 95% confidence interval for the population proportion is:[2]

$\{[p - 2 \times SE(p)]$ to $[p + 2 \times SE(p)]\}.$

For example, in Table 1.2 the percentage of cases (those women with a malignant diagnosis) who are pre-menopausal is 13%, so the sample proportion p is 0.13, and:

$$SE(p) = \sqrt{\frac{0.13(1 - 0.13)}{106}} = 0.033.$$

Therefore the 95% confidence interval for the population proportion is:

$(0.13 - 2 \times 0.033)$ to $(0.13 + 2 \times 0.033) = (0.064$ to $0.196).$

In other words, you can be 95% confident that somewhere in the interval from 0.064 to 0.196 (or 6.4% to 19.6%) will be found the population proportion (percentage) of cases who are pre-menopausal. Alternatively, this interval represents a plausible range of values for the population proportion.

Exercise 9.4
Calculate the standard error for the proportion of controls in Table 1.2 who are pre-menopausal, and hence calculate the 95% confidence interval for this proportion. Interpret your result.

---

[2] I use the value 2 in the following expression, but the exact value is 1.96.

An Example from Practice

Table 9.2 is from a randomised controlled trial to test the short-term efficacy of a self-directed treatment manual for bulimia nervosa. There were three randomised groups: those given the manual, those given cognitive behavioural therapy, and those simply allocated to a waiting list. The figure shows the proportion in each group abstaining from a number of troubling behaviours at the end of the study, along with the 95% confidence intervals.

Table 9.2 Sample percentages of patients in each of three groups abstaining from a number of troubling diet-related behaviours by the end of the study, along with the 95% confidence intervals for the corresponding population percentages

VARIABLE	MANUAL (No [%], 95% confidence interval†)	COGNITIVE BEHAVIOURAL THERAPY (No [%], 95% confidence interval†)	WAITING LIST (No [%], 95% confidence interval†)	χ^2 (2 df)
Binge eating*	11/35 (31%), 14 to 45%	7/20 (35%), 16 to 62%	3/19 (17%), 13 to 40%	1.79, p = 0.41
Vomiting*	7/29 (24%), 8 to 40%	4/14 (29%), 8 to 58%	2/13 (15%), 5 to 51%	0.69, p = 0.71
Other weight-control behaviours*	12/19 (63%), 36 to 81%	5/8 (62%), 18 to 90%	1/8 (12%), 0.3 to 53%	6.29, p = ≤0.05
Full remission	9/41 (22%), 9 to 34%	5/21 (24%), 8 to 47%	2/19 (11%), 1 to 32%	1.36, p = 0.51

*Only patients who engaged in these behaviours at first assessment but who were abstinent at second assessment have been included.
†95% confidence interval for proportion of abstinence.

The sample percentage of subjects in the manual group who had abstained from binge eating at the end of the study was 31% (11 subjects out of 35), so the sample proportion is 0.31, and SE(p) = √[0.31(1 − 0.31)/35] = √0.0061 = 0.078. The 95% confidence interval is therefore (0.31 − 2 × 0.078) to (0.31 + 2 × 0.078) = (0.154 to 0.466). As you can see, this is the same result as shown in the table. You can be 95% confident that this interval will contain the population proportion or percentage abstaining from binge eating.

Exercise 9.5
Interpret and compare the sample percentages and their respective confidence intervals, for the percentage in each group in Table 9.2 who had abstained from vomiting by the end of the study.

ESTIMATING A CONFIDENCE INTERVAL FOR THE MEDIAN OF A SINGLE POPULATION

If your data is ordinal, the median rather than the mean is the appropriate measure of location (review Chapters 1 and 5 if you're not sure why). Alternatively, if your data is metric but skewed (or your sample is too small to check the distributional shape), you might also prefer the median as a more representative measure. Either way, a confidence interval will enable you to assess the likely range of values for the population median. SPSS does not calculate a confidence interval for a single median, but Minitab does and bases its calculation on the Wilcoxon signed-rank procedure (I'll discuss this in Chapter 12).

An Example from Practice

Table 9.3 is from the analgesics and stump pain study referred to in Table 5.3 and shows the sample median pain levels and their 95% confidence intervals (assessed using a visual analogue scale), for the treatment and control groups, at three time periods.

Table 9.3   Sample median pain levels, and 95% confidence intervals for the difference between the two groups, at three time periods, in the analgesics/stump pain study

	MEDIAN (IQR) PAIN		
	Blockade group (n = 27)	Control group (n = 29)	95% CI for difference (p)
After epidural bolus	0 (0–0)	38 (17–67)	24 to 43 (p <0.0001)
After continuous epidural infusion	0 (0–0)	31 (20–51)	24 to 43 (p <0.0001)
After epidural bolus in operating theatre	0 (0–0)	35 (16–64)	19 to 42 (p <0.0001)

Pain assessed by visual analogue scale (0–100mm).

Exercise 9.6
In Table 9.3, interpret and compare the differences in median pain levels and their 95% confidence intervals, for each of the three time periods.

10

ESTIMATING THE DIFFERENCE BETWEEN *TWO* POPULATION PARAMETERS

Learning objectives

When you have finished this chapter you should be able to:

- *Give some examples of situations where there is a need to estimate the difference between two population parameters*
- *Interpret results from studies which estimate the difference between two population means, two percentages, or two medians, either matched or independent*
- *Demonstrate an awareness of any assumptions which must be satisfied when estimating the difference between two population parameters*

What's the Difference?

As you saw in Chapter 9, it's possible to determine confidence intervals for any single population parameter—means, medians, percentages, etc., but by far the most common application is the comparison of some population parameter in *two* groups, in particular between two population *means*. I'll start with this.

ESTIMATING THE DIFFERENCE BETWEEN THE *MEANS* OF *TWO INDEPENDENT* POPULATIONS

The procedure here, like that for the single mean (see Chapter 9), is based on the *t*-distribution. With *two* populations, you need to know whether if they are *matched* or *independent*, since this affects the analysis (see page 69 to review matching). I'll start with *independent* populations. There are a number of assumptions which need to be met if you want to calculate a confidence interval for the difference between two independent population means.

Assumptions

- Data for both groups must be *metric*. As you know from Chapter 5, the mean is appropriate only with metric data anyway.

- The distribution of the relevant variable in each population must be reasonably *Normal*. You can check this assumption from the sample data using a histogram, although with small sample sizes this can be difficult.
- The population standard deviations of the two variables concerned should be *approximately* the same, but this requirement becomes less important as sample sizes get larger. You can check this using the sample standard deviations, but Minitab and SPSS provide alternative analyses for both equal and unequal standard deviations. Minitab asks you to specify whether standard deviations are equal or not, SPSS calculates confidence intervals for both situations.

An Example using Birthweights

Suppose you want to compare the population mean birthweights (i.e. estimate the difference between them) of the 30 infants born in a maternity unit (data in Table 2.1), with that of 30 infants born at home (data in Table 10.1). The two samples are selected independently with no attempt at matching.

Both SPSS and Minitab compute the sample mean birthweight of the home-born infants to be 3726.5g, with a standard deviation of 385.7g. Recall from p. 55 that for the infants born in the maternity units, sample mean birthweight was 3644.4g with a standard deviation of 376.8g. So there *is* a difference in the *sample* mean birthweights of 3726.5 minus 3644.4 = 82.1g, but this does *not* mean that there is a difference in the *population* mean birthweights—this sample difference might simply be due to chance.

Now we come to an important point:

> If the 95% confidence interval for the difference between two population parameters includes 0, then you can be 95% confident that there is no difference in their values.

After all, if 0 is a possible value, then you can't exclude the possibility that 0 *is* the value. In other words, if you want to know whether there is a statistically significant difference between two population means, calculate the 95% confidence interval for the difference and see whether it contains 0. If it *doesn't* you can be 95% confident that there *is* a statistically significant difference in the means. If it does, assume there is *no* statistically significant difference, and the difference between the two sample means is due purely to chance. It is possible to calculate these confidence intervals by hand but the process is time-consuming and tedious; fortunately, as usual, most statistics programs will do the sums for you. Since differences between independent population means is one of the most commonly used procedures in clinical research, you might find it helpful to see some output from SPSS and Minitab for this procedure.

With SPSS
Using the birthweight data in Table 10.1, SPSS produces the results (with some material deleted) shown in Figure 10.1. The output tells us that the difference in the two *sample* mean birthweights is 82.17g. The sign in front of this value

Table 10.1 Sample data for birthweight (g), Apgar scores, and whether mother smoked during pregnancy, for 30 infants born in a maternity unit and at home

INFANT	BIRTHWEIGHT (g)		MOTHER SMOKED*		APGAR SCORE	
	Hospital birth	*Home birth*	*Hospital birth*	*Home birth*	*Hospital birth*	*Home birth*
1	3710	3810	0	0	8	10
2	3650	3865	0	0	7	8
3	4490	. 4578	0	0	8	9
4	3421	3522	1	0	6	6
5	3399	3400	0	1	6	7
6	4094	4156	0	0	9	10
7	4006	4200	0	0	8	9
8	3287	3265	1	0	5	6
9	3594	3599	0	1	7	8
10	4206	4215	0	0	9	10
11	3508	3697	0	0	7	8
12	4010	4209	0	0	8	9
13	3896	3911	0	0	8	8
14	3800	3943	0	0	8	9
15	2860	3000	0	1	4	3
16	3798	3802	0	0	8	9
17	3666	3654	0	0	7	8
18	4200	4295	1	0	9	10
19	3615	3732	0	0	7	8
20	3193	3098	1	1	4	5
21	2994	3105	1	1	5	5
22	3266	3455	1	0	5	6
23	3400	3507	0	0	6	7
24	4090	4103	0	0	8	9
25	3303	3456	1	0	6	7
26	3447	3538	1	0	6	7
27	3388	3400	1	1	6	7
28	3613	3715	0	0	7	7
29	3541	3566	0	0	7	8
30	3886	4000	1	0	8	6

* 0 = no, 1 = yes

depends on which variable you select first in the SPSS dialogue box. SPSS subtracts the second variable selected (maternity unit births) from the first (home births), so this result means that the sample mean birthweight was 82.17g higher in the home-birth infants.

SPSS calculates two confidence intervals, one with standard deviations assumed to be equal, and one with them not equal.[1] The 95% confidence interval shown in the last two columns is (−114.9g to 279.2g), and is the same in both cases. SPSS tests for equality of the standard deviations (variances) using Levene's test. We will look at tests in Chapter 12, but all you need to know for now is that the working assumption is that the two population standard deviations *are* equal. If the value in the column headed "Levene's Test for Equality of Variances—Sig." is

[1] Both Minitab and SPSS refer to equality of *variances.* Variances is equal to standard deviation squared.

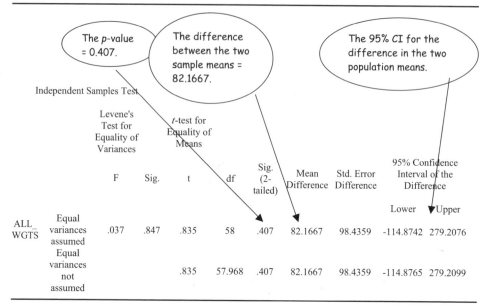

		Levene's Test for Equality of Variances		*t*-test for Equality of Means					95% Confidence Interval of the Difference	
		F	Sig.	t	df	Sig. (2-tailed)	Mean Difference	Std. Error Difference	Lower	Upper
ALL WGTS	Equal variances assumed	.037	.847	.835	58	.407	82.1667	98.4359	-114.8742	279.2076
	Equal variances not assumed			.835	57.968	.407	82.1667	98.4359	-114.8765	279.2099

Figure 10.1: SPSS output for the 95% confidence interval (last two columns) for the difference between two independent population mean birthweights, using samples of 30 infants born in maternity units and 30 at home. Data in Tables 2.1 and 10.1

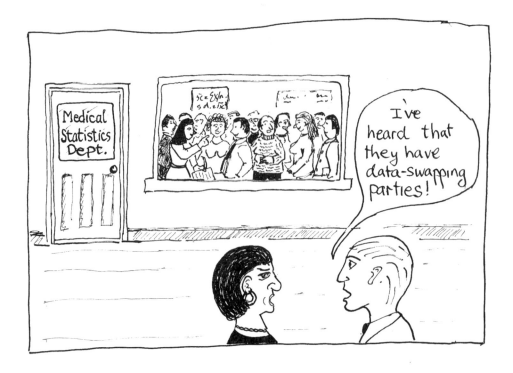

equal to or greater than 0.05, then this assumption is confirmed; otherwise not. In this case the value is 0.847, which is more than 0.05, so the standard deviations are the same. This is not really surprising since the sample standard deviations are so alike. Since this confidence interval includes 0, you can conclude that there is no statistically significant difference in *population* mean birthweights of infants born in the maternity unit and at home.   CI includes 0   SD = same

With Minitab

The Minitab output, which confirms that from SPSS, is shown in Figure 10.2. The 95% confidence interval is in the second row up.

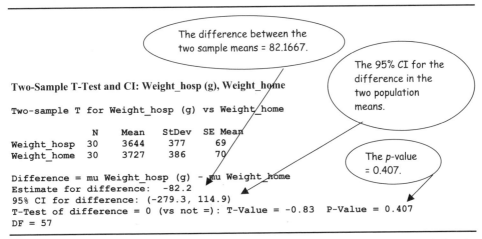

Figure 10.2: Minitab output for the 95% confidence interval (second row up) for the difference between two independent population mean birthweights, using samples of 30 infants born in maternity units and 30 at home

An Example from Practice

Table 10.2 is from a cohort study of maternal smoking during pregnancy, and infant growth after birth. The subjects were 12,987 babies who were followed-up for three years after birth. Of these, 10,238 had non-smoking mothers, 2276 had mothers who had smoked one to nine cigarettes a day, and 473 had mothers who had smoked 10 or more cigarettes a day. The figure shows the 95% confidence intervals for differences in mean weight according to sex of baby and smoking habits of mothers, at birth, at 3 months, and at 6 months.

The results show, for example, that at birth, the difference between the sample mean weight of female babies born to non-smoking mothers, and those born to mothers smoking 10 or more cigarettes a day, was 3220 minus 3052 = 168g. That is, the infants of smoking mothers are on average lighter by 168g. Is this difference statistically significant in the population, or due simply to chance? The 95% confidence interval of (−234 to −102)g does *not* include 0, so you can be 95% confident that the difference is real (i.e. is statistically significant).

Table 10.2 95% confidence intervals for difference in weights according to sex and smoking habits of mothers between independent groups of babies, according to sex and smoking habit of mother, at birth, 3 months, and 6 months

MOTHER'S SMOKING HABIT	AT BIRTH			AT 3 MONTHS			AT 6 MONTHS		
	No.	Weight	95% confidence interval for difference	No.	Weight	95% confidence interval for difference	No.	Weight	95% confidence interval for difference
Girls:									
Non-smokers	4904	3220		4904	5584		4895	7462	
1–9 Cigarettes/day	1072	3132	(–121 to –55)	1071	5550	(–77 to 9)	1072	7471	(–47 to 65)
≥10 Cigarettes/day	228	3052	(–234 to –102)	228	5519	(–152 to 22)	227	7434	(–141 to 85)
Boys									
Non-smokers	5334	3373		5332	6026		5330	8038	
1–9 Cigarettes/day	1204	3266	(–139 to –75)	1204	5958	(–113 to –23)	1204	7974	(–118 to –10)
≥10 Cigarettes/daily	245	3126	(–312 to –181)	245	5907	(–212 to –26)	245	8014	(–136 to 88)

Exercise 10.1

Interpret the sample mean and confidence intervals for all four differences in weights at 6 months.

ESTIMATING THE DIFFERENCE BETWEEN TWO *MATCHED* POPULATION MEANS

If you investigate the difference between individuals in two groups, let's say in birthweight, you are interested in how much average birthweight differs or *varies between* the two groups, not in how much birthweights vary *within* the individuals belonging to either one of the groups.[2] In fact the latter differences get in the way, particularly if the variation within the groups is large, and may obscure any real differences between the group averages. This is illustrated in Figure 10.3.

When data is matched (see Chapter 6 for an explanation of matching), this reduces much of the within-group variation, and for a given sample size makes it easier to detect differences between groups. This means you can achieve better precision (narrower confidence intervals), without having to increase sample size. The disadvantage of matching is that it is sometimes difficult to find a sufficiently large number of matches (as you saw in the case–control discussion earlier).

In the independent groups case above, the mean of each group is computed separately, and then a confidence interval for the difference in these means is calculated. In the matched groups case, the difference between each pair of values is computed, and then a confidence interval for the mean of these *differences* is calculated.

An Example from Practice

Table 10.3 shows the 95% confidence intervals for the difference in bone mineral density in two individually matched groups of women, one group depressed and one "normal".

---

[2] Known as *between-group* and *within-group* variation, respectively.

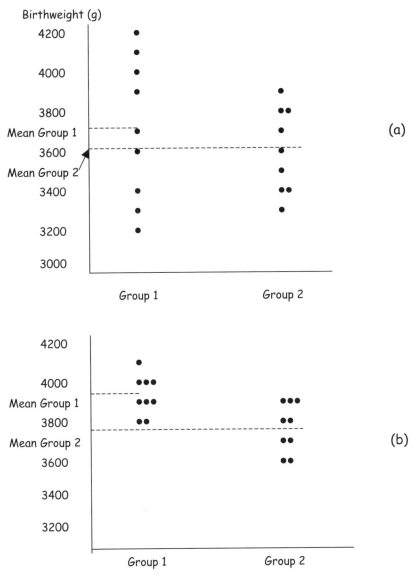

Figure 10.3: In (a) and (b) the difference in the mean birthweights between the two groups is similar. However, in (a) the fact that *within* group 1 there is a wide variation in birthweight makes it difficult to detect this difference in means. In (b), the variation within each group is smaller, making it much easier to detect that there is a difference *between* the two means

(Ignore the "SD from expected peak" rows.) Only one of the confidence intervals contains 0, indicating that there is no difference in population mean bone mineral density at the radius, but there is at all of the other five sites.

Exercise 10.2
Which population difference in bone mineral density in Table 10.3 is estimated with the greatest precision?

Table 10.3   Confidence intervals for the differences between the population mean bone mineral densities in two individually *matched* groups of women, one group depressed, the other "normal"

BONE MEASURED†	DEPRESSED WOMEN	NORMAL WOMEN	MEAN DIFFERENCE (95% CI)	p VALUE
Lumbar spine (anteroposterior)				
Density (g/cm²)	1.00±0.15	1.07±0.09	0.08 (0.02 to 0.14)	0.02
SD from expected peak	−0.42±1.28	0.26±0.82	0.68 (0.13 to 1.23)	
Lumbar spine (lateral)‡				
Density (g/cm²)	0.74±0.09	0.79±0.07	0.05 (0.00 to 0.09)	0.03
SD from expected peak	−0.88±1.07	−0.36±0.80	0.50 (0.04 to 1.03)	
Femoral neck				
Density (g/cm²)	0.76±0.11	0.88±0.11	0.11 (0.06 to 0.17)	<0.001
SD from expected peak	−1.30±1.07	−0.22±0.99	1.08 (0.55 to 1.61)	
Ward's triangle				
Density (g/cm²)	0.70±0.14	0.81±0.13	0.11 (0.06 to 0.17)	<0.00
SD from expected peak	−0.93±1.24	0.18±1.22	1.11 (0.60 to 1.62)	
Trochanter				
Density (g/cm²)	0.66±0.11	0.74±0.08	0.08 (0.04 to 0.13)	<0.001
SD from expected peak	−0.70±1.22	0.26±0.91	0.97 (0.46 to 1.47)	
Radius				
Density (g/cm²)	0.68±0.04	0.70±0.04	0.01 (−0.01 to 0.04)	0.25
SD from expected peak	−0.19±0.67	0.03±0.67	0.21 (−0.21 to 0.64)	

*Plus−minus values are means ±SD. CI denotes confidence interval.
†Values for "SD from expected peak" are the numbers of standard deviations from the expected peak density derived from a population-based study of normal white women.
‡This measurement was made in 23 depressed women and 23 normal women.

ESTIMATING THE DIFFERENCE BETWEEN TWO *INDEPENDENT* POPULATION PERCENTAGES

Suppose you want to calculate a 95% confidence interval for the difference between the percentage of women having maternity unit births who smoked during pregnancy, and the percentage having home births who smoked. The data on smoking status for the 60 mothers is shown in Table 10.1. There are 10 mothers among the 30 giving birth in the maternity unit, and six among the 30 giving birth at home, who smoked. This gives proportions of 10/30 = 0.3333, or 33.33%, and 6/30 = 0.2000, or 20%, respectively.

However, you could have got the same results by calculating the *mean* of each column (look back to Table 5.1). So with binary data the difference in percentages is equivalent to the difference in means, and the same two-sample *t*-procedure, or the matched-pairs *t*-procedure, described there can be used. The *sample* evidence in the childbirth example above suggests that there may be a statistically significant difference in the percentages, but the result could be due entirely to chance. A confidence interval would help you decide which.

ESTIMATING THE DIFFERENCE BETWEEN TWO *MATCHED* POPULATION PERCENTAGES

With individually matched subjects you can use the same approach as for the matched means described above. The matching has the same effect as before, suppression of within-group variation providing narrower, more precise confidence intervals for the same sample size.

ESTIMATING THE DIFFERENCE BETWEEN TWO *INDEPENDENT* POPULATION MEDIANS

As you know from Chapter 5, the mean may not be the most representative measure of location if the data is skewed, and is not appropriate anyway if the data is ordinal. In these circumstances you can instead compare the population *medians*, and instead of the two-sample *t*-procedure, use a *non-parametric* equivalent, the *Mann–Whitney* procedure, to do this. A *parametric* procedure can only be applied to data which is metric and follows some particular distribution, often the Normal distribution. However, if your data has neither of these properties, for example if it is ordinal, you can use a non-parametric procedure which does not make these requirements of the data. Mann–Whitney only requires that the two population distributions have the same approximate shape, but does not require it to be Normal.

Briefly, the Mann–Whitney procedure starts by combining the data from both groups, which are then ranked. The rank values for each group are then separated and summed. If the medians of the two groups are the same then the rank sums of the two groups should be similar. So if the sample rank sums are different, you need to know whether this difference is due to chance or because there is a real statistically significant difference in the population medians. A Mann–Whitney confidence interval for the difference in the rank sums will help you decide which.

As an illustration, let's compare the difference in the population median Apgar scores for the maternity unit and home-birth infants, using the data in Table 10.1. The output from Minitab is shown in Figure 10.4, with the 95% confidence interval in the fourth row.[3] Since the confidence interval of (–2 to 0) contains 0,

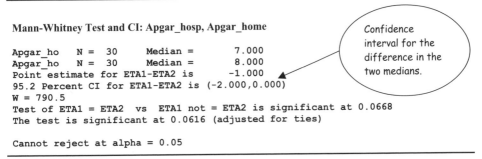

Figure 10.4:   Minitab output for a 95% confidence interval for the difference between two independent median Apgar scores, for infants born in maternity units and at home (raw data in Table 10.1)

---

[3] SPSS does not appear to calculate a confidence interval for two independent medians.

you conclude that the difference in the population median Apgar scores is not statistically significant. Notice that the confidence level is given as 95.2%, not 95%. Confidence intervals for medians cannot always achieve the precise confidence level you stipulated, because of the way in which a median is calculated.

An Example from Practice

Table 10.4 is from a randomised controlled double-blind trial in an A&E department to compare the cost-effectiveness of ketorolac versus morphine, in relieving pain after blunt instrument injury. The penultimate column contains the 95% confidence intervals for the difference in various median treatment times (minutes), between the ketorolac and morphine groups (ignore the last column). As the footnote to the table indicates, these results were obtained using the Mann–Whitney procedure.

Table 10.4 Confidence intervals for the difference between two *independent* population medians (times in minutes) relating to patients' treatment. One group received ketorolac, the other morphine. Taken from a randomised controlled double-blind trial comparing the cost-effectiveness of intravenous ketorolac versus intravenous morphine in relieving pain after blunt instrument injury in an A&E department

VARIABLE	KETOROLAC GROUP (n = 75)	MORPHINE GROUP (n = 73)	MEDIAN DIFFERENCE (95% confidence interval)	p-VALUE*
Interval between arrival in emergency department and doctor prescribing analgesia	38.0 (30.0 to 54.0)	39.0 (29.0 to 53.0)	1.0 (−5.0 to 7.0)	0.72
Preparation for analgesia	5.0 (5.0 to 10.0)	10.0 (5.5 to 12.5)	2.0 (0 to 5.0)	0.0002
Undergoing radiography	5.0 (5.0 to 10.0)	5.0 (4.0 to 10.0)	0 (−1.0 to 0)	0.75
Total time spent in emergency department	155.0 (112.0 to 198.0)	171.0 (126.0 to 208.5)	15.0 (−4.0 to 33.0)	0.11
Interval between receiving analgesia and leaving emergency department	155.0 (75.0 to 149.0)	130.0 (95.0 to 170.0)	20.0 (4.0 to 39.0)	0.02

Mann-Whitney test

The only confidence interval not containing 0 is that for the difference in median "interval between receiving analgesia and leaving A&E", for which the difference in the sample medians is 20.0 minutes. So this is the only treatment time for which the difference in population median times is statistically significant, and you can be 95% confident that this difference is between 4 and 39 minutes.

Exercise 10.3
Table 10.4 includes the sample median times and their 95% confidence intervals for each time interval, for both groups separately. Only one pair of confidence intervals don't

overlap, those for the only time difference which is statistically significant. Why aren't you surprised by this?

ESTIMATING THE DIFFERENCE BETWEEN TWO *MATCHED* POPULATION MEDIANS

When two groups are matched, but either the data is ordinal, or if metric is noticeably skewed, you can obtain confidence intervals for differences in population medians, using the non-parametric *Wilcoxon* procedure. There are no distributional requirements, but the two population distributions, regardless of shape, should be symmetric. This is the non-parametric equivalent of the parametric matched-pairs *t*-procedure, described above. The matching will again reduce the variation within groups, so narrower, and therefore more precise confidence intervals are available for a given sample size.

Briefly the Wilcoxon procedure starts by calculating the difference between each pair of values, and these differences are then ranked (ignoring any minus signs). Any negative signs are then restored to the ranks, and the negative and positive ranks are separately summed. If the medians in the two groups are the same, then these two rank sums should be similar. If different, the Wilcoxon procedure provides a way of determining whether this is due to chance or represents a statistically significant difference in the population medians.

SPSS does not provide this confidence interval calculation. To get Minitab to apply a Wilcoxon procedure you have to use Minitab's Calculate facility first to calculate the differences between each pair of scores. The procedure is then applied to this single column of difference values.

An Example from Practice

Table 10.5 contains the results of a case–control study into the dietary intake of schizophrenic patients living in the community in Scotland (ignore the last column), and shows the daily energy intake of eight dietary substances for the cases (17 men and 13 women diagnosed with schizophrenia), and the controls, each individually matched on sex, age, smoking status, and employment status.

If you focus on the penultimate column, in which data for men and women is combined, you can see that only the confidence interval for daily protein intake, (−1.1g to 32.8g), contains 0, which implies that there is no difference in population median protein intake between schizophrenics and normal individuals. For all other substances the difference is statistically significant.

Exercise 10.4
Explain the meaning of the 95% confidence interval for difference in median alcohol intake of the two groups in Table 10.5.

Table 10.5 Results from a matched case–control study of the dietary habits of schizophrenics, showing confidence intervals for the difference in population median food intakes per day for a number of substances. Values are median (range)

INTAKE DAY	MEN		WOMEN		ALL		WILCOXON SIGNED RANKS TEST	
	Patients (n = 17)	Controls (n = 17)	Patients (n = 13)	Controls (n = 13)	Patients (n = 30)	Controls (n = 30)	Median difference (95% CI)	P
Energy (MJ)	11.84 (7.67–17.93)	14.19 (6.94–23.22)	8.87 (5.07–13.02)	9.99 (5.25–16.25)	9.71 (5.07–17.94)	11.98 (5.25–23.22)	2.06 (0.26–4.23)	0.04
Protein (g)	92.5 (65.1–157.4)	114.2 (74–633)	68.7 (38.4–104.2)	82.5 (40.5–142.2)	84.5 (38.4–157.4)	96.0 (40.5–633.0)	15.9 (–1.1 to 32.8)	0.07
Total fibre (g)	13.0 (8.5–20.8)	22.0 (8.7–86.2)	10.7 (7.3–18.0)	15.5 (10.7–22.9)	12.6 (7.3–20.8)	18.9 (8.7–86.2)	7.0 (3.6 to 10.6)	0.0001
Retinol (µg)	647 (294–1498)	817 (134–12 341)	533 (288–7556)	817 (201–11 585)	590 (288–7556)	817 (134–12 341)	310 (93 to 1269)	0.02
Carotene (µg)	783 (219–3638)	2510 (523–11 313)	2048 (550–4657)	3079 (956–6188)	1443 (219–4657)	2798 (523–11 313)	1376 (549 to 2452)	0.004
Vitamin C (mg)	41.0 (4.0–204)	81.0 (14.0–262)	40.0 (3–165)	61.0 (27.0–291.0)	40.5 (3.0–204)	80.5 (14.0–219)	33.5 (2.0 to 64.0)	0.03
Vitamin E (mg)	4.8 (3.4–18.0)	10.26 (2.23–32.0)	4.5 (2.3–6.0)	5.38 (3.6–14.7)	4.7 (2.3–18.0)	7.8 (2.2–32.0)	2.9 (1.45 to 5.35)	0.0002
Alcohol (g)	3.8 (0–19.4)	11.7 (0–80)	0 (0–5.5)	1.8 (0–12)	0 (0–19.4)	5.7 (0–80)	5.4 (1.2 to 9.9)	0.009

11

ESTIMATING THE *RATIO* OF TWO POPULATION PARAMETERS

Learning objectives

When you have finished this chapter you should be able to:

- *Explain what is meant by the ratio of two population parameters and give some examples of situations where there is a need to estimate such a ratio*
- *Explain and interpret a confidence interval for a risk radio*
- *Explain and interpret a confidence interval for an odds ratio*
- *Explain the difference between crude and adjusted risk and odds ratios*

Ratios

Suppose the mean parity in one population of women is 3.5, and in a second population is 2.0; then the *ratio* of the first mean to the second mean is equal to 3.5 to 2.0, or 1.75 to 1 (dividing the first number by the second). In other words the first mean is 75% bigger than, or 1.75 times, the second mean. In practice you can write the ratio as just 1.75, the "to 1" is understood.

To state the blindingly obvious, if the two numbers have the same value, their ratio is equal to 1. Conversely, if the ratio of any two numbers is 1, then you know that they're equal. You can use this idea to calculate and interpret confidence interval estimates of the *ratio* of two population parameters.

ESTIMATING THE RATIO OF TWO INDEPENDENT POPULATION MEANS

When you compare two *population* means you usually want to know whether they're the same, and if not, how big the difference between them is. Sometimes though, you might want to know *how many times bigger* one population mean is than another. The ratio of the two means will tell you that. If two sample means have a ratio of 1, this tells us *only* that the means are the same size in the *sample*. If the sample ratio *is* different from 1, you need to check whether this is a statistically significant difference, implying that one population mean *is* bigger than the other, or is simply due to chance. You can do this with a 95% confidence interval for the population ratio. And here's the rule:

> If the confidence interval for the *ratio* of two population parameters does *not* contain the value 1, then you can be 95% confident that any difference in the size of the two measures is statistically significant.

Compare this with the rule for the *difference* between two population parameters, where the rule is that if the confidence interval does *not* contain *0*, then any difference between the two parameters *is* statistically significant.

An Example from Practice

Look again at the last column in Table 9.1, which shows a number of outputs from a randomised trial to compare integrated versus conventional care for asthma patients. The last column contains the 95% confidence intervals for the ratio of population means for the treatment and control groups, for a number of outcomes. You will see that *all* of the confidence intervals contain 1, indicating that the population mean number of bronchodilators used, the number of inhaled steroids prescribed, and so on, was no larger (or smaller) in one population than in the other.

The *sample* ratio furthest away from 1 is 1.31, for the ratio of mean number of hospital admissions; that is, the *sample* of integrated care group patients had 31% more admissions than the conventionally treated control group patients. However, the 95% confidence interval of (0.87 to 1.96) includes 1, which implies that this is *not* the case in the populations.

CONFIDENCE INTERVALS FOR A POPULATION RISK RATIO

Look back at Table 6.1 which shows the contingency table for a cohort study into the risk of coronary heart disease (CHD) as an adult, among men who weighed less than 18lb at 12 months old. On page 91 we derived a risk ratio of 1.93 from this sample cohort. In other words, men who weighed less than 18lb at one year appear, as an adult, to have nearly twice the risk of CHD as men who weighed 18lb or more at one year. But is this true in the population of such men, or no more than a *chance* departure from a population ratio of 1? You now know that you can answer this question by examining the 95% confidence interval for this risk ratio.

The 95% confidence interval for the CHD risk ratio turns out to be (0.793 to 4.697). Since this interval contains 1 you can conclude, despite a *sample* risk ratio of nearly 2, that weighing less than 18lb at one year is *not* a risk factor for coronary heart disease in adult life in the sampled *population*. Notice that, in general, the value of a sample risk or odds ratio, as in this example, does *not* lie in the centre of its confidence interval, but is usually closer to the lower value.

An Example from Practice

Table 11.1 is from a cohort study of 552 men surviving acute myocardial infarction, in which each subject was assessed for depression at the beginning of the study: 14.5% were identified as severely depressed, 2.3% as moderately depressed, and 63.2% had low levels of depression. The subjects were followed-up at 6 months, and a number of outcomes measured—including suffering angina, returning to work, emotional stability, and smoking. The researchers were interested in examining the role of moderate and of severe depression (compared to low depression) as risk factors for each of these outcomes.

Table 11.1 Crude and adjusted risk ratios for a number of outcomes related to the risk of moderate and severe levels of depression compared to low depression, 6 months after a myocardial infarction in a cohort study of 552 males

DEPRESSION LEVEL	RELATIVE RISK (95% CI)		STANDARDISED REGRESSION COEFFICIENT
	Crude	*Adjusted‡*	*Adjusted*
Angina pectoris†			
Moderate	1.36 (0.83 to 2.23)	0.97 (0.55 to 1.70)	−0.008
Severe	3.12 (1.58 to 6.16)	2.31 (1.11 to 4.80)	0.158
Return to work			
Moderate	0.41 (0.22 to 0.77)	0.58 (0.28 to 1.17)	−0.127
Severe	0.39 (0.18 to 0.88)	0.54 (0.22 to 1.31)	−0.116
Emotional instability‡			
Moderate	2.21 (1.33 to 3.69)	1.87 (1.07 to 3.27)	0.143
Severe	5.55 (2.87 to 10.71)	4.61 (2.32 to 9.18)	0.288
Smoking			
Moderate	1.39 (0.71 to 2.73)	1.19 (0.56 to 2.51)	0.040
Severe	2.63 (1.23 to 5.60)	2.84 (1.22 to 6.63)	0.201
Late potential§			
Moderate	1.30 (0.76 to 2.22)	1.54 (0.86 to 2.74)	0.099
Severe	0.70 (0.33 to 1.47)	0.75 (0.35 to 2.17)	−0.054

*For angina pectoris, the adherence to anti-anginal medication and the presence of pre-AMI angina were added to the logistic regression model.
†Angina pectoris during low or high exertion or at rest; ‡Zung self-rating-anxiety scale; §duration of prolonged QRS ≥120ms or V (40ms) <25µV using a 25Hz high-pass filter.
‡Adjusted for age, social class, recurrent infarction, rehabilitation, cardiac events and helplessness.

The results show the crude and adjusted risk ratios (labelled "relative risk" by the authors) for each outcome. The crude risk ratios are *not* adjusted for any confounding factors, whereas the adjusted risk ratios *are* adjusted, for the factors listed in the table footnote (review the material on confounding and adjustment in Chapter 6 if necessary).

Let's interpret the 95% risk ratios for "Return to work". The *crude* risk ratios for a return to work indicate lower rates of return to work for men both moderately depressed (risk ratio = 0.41) and severely depressed (risk ratio = 0.39), compared to men with low levels of depression. Neither of the confidence intervals, (0.22 to 0.77) and (0.18 to 0.88), includes 1. However, after adjusting for possible confounding variables, the *adjusted* risk ratios are 0.58 and 0.54, and are no longer statistically significant, because the confidence intervals for both risk ratios, for moderate depression (0.28 to 1.17), and severe depression (0.22 to 1.31), now include 1.

Exercise 11.1

Table 11.2 is from the same cohort study referred to in Exercise 8.9, to investigate dental disease and risk of coronary heart disease (CHD), and mortality, involving over 20,000 men and women aged 25–74, who were followed up between 1971–74 and 1986–87. Dental disease, CHD and mortality were recorded. The results give the risk ratios (called "relative risks" here) for CHD and for mortality in those with a number of dental diseases, compared to those without dental disease (the referent group), and adjusted for a number of other variables (see the table footnote for a list of the variables adjusted for). Briefly summarise what the results show about dental disease as a risk factor for CHD and mortality. Note: the periodontal index, range from 0 to 8 (higher is worse), measures the average degree of periodontal disease in all teeth present, and the oral hygiene indexes (range 0–6, higher is worse) measures the average degree of debris and calculus on the surfaces of six selected teeth.

Table 11.2 Adjusted* risk ratios (and 95% confidence intervals) for CDH and mortality among those with dental disease compared to those without dental disease

INDICATOR	NO. OF SUBJECTS†	CORONARY HEART DISEASE	TOTAL MORTALITY
Peridontal class			
No disease	673	1.00	1.00
Gingivitis	529	0.98 (0.63 to 1.54)	1.42 (0.84 to 2.42)
Periodontitis	300	1.72 (1.10 to 2.68)	2.12 (1.24 to 3.62)
No teeth	92	1.71 (0.93 to 3.15)	2.60 (1.33 to 5.07)
Peridontal index (per unit)	1502	1.09 (1.00 to 1.19)	1.11 (0.01 to 1.22)
Oral hygiene (per unit)	1436	1.11 (0.96 to 1.27)	1.23 (1.06 to 1.43)

*Adjusted for age, sex, race, education, poverty index, marital state, systolic blood pressure, total cholesterol concentration, diabetes, body mass index, physical activity, alcohol consumption, and cigarette smoking.
†Excluding those with missing data for any variable and, for periodontal index and hygiene index, those who had no teeth.

CONFIDENCE INTERVALS FOR A POPULATION ODDS RATIO

Table 6.2 showed the data for the case–control study into exercise between the ages of 15 and 25 and stroke later in life. The risk factor here is "not exercising", and we calculated the *sample* crude odds ratio for a stroke in those who hadn't exercised compared to those who had, as 0.411 (see page 92). So the exercising group appear to have under half the odds for a stroke as the non-exercising group. However, you need to examine the confidence interval for this odds ratio to see whether it contains 1 or not, before you can come to a conclusion about the statistically significance of the *population* odds ratio.

SPSS produces an odds ratio of 0.411, with a 95% confidence interval of (0.260 to 0.650). This does not contain 1, so you can be 95% confident that the odds ratio for a stroke in the *population* of those who did exercise compared to the population of those who didn't exercise is somewhere between 0.260 and 0.650. So early-life exercise does seem to reduce the odds for a stroke later on. Of course this is a crude, unadjusted odds ratio, which takes no account of the contribution, positive or negative, of any other relevant variables.

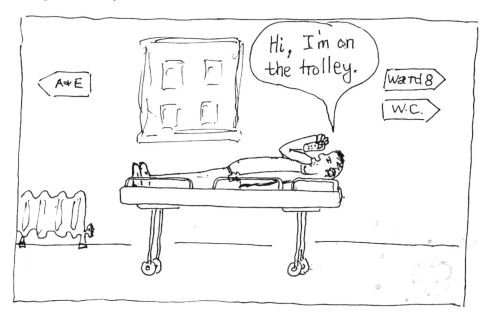

An Example from Practice

Table 11.3 shows the results from this same case–control study, where the authors provide both crude odds ratios, and ratios *adjusted* for age and sex.

Table 11.3 Crude and adjusted odds ratios for stroke patients according to whether and at what age exercise was undertaken by patients compared to controls without stroke

AGE WHEN EXERCISE UNDERTAKEN (years):	EXERCISE NOT UNDERTAKEN		EXERCISE UNDERTAKEN	
	Odds ratio	*No. of cases: no. of controls*	*Odds ratio (95% confidence interval)*	*No. of cases: no. of controls*
15–25	1.0	70:68	0.33 (0.2 to 0.6)	55:130
25–40	1.0	103:136	0.43 (0.2 to 0.8)	21:57
40–55	1.0	101:139	0.63 (0.3 to 1.5)	10:22

We have been looking at exercise between the ages of 15 and 25, the first row of the table. Compared to the *crude* odds ratio calculated above of 0.411, the authors report an odds ratio for stroke, *adjusted* for age and sex, among those who exercised compared to those who didn't exercise as 0.33 with a 95% confidence interval of (0.20 to 0.60). So even after the effects of any differences in age and sex between the two groups have been adjusted for, exercising remains a statistically significant risk factor for stroke (although beneficial in this case). Adjustment for possible confounders is crucial if your results are to be of any use, and I will return to adjustment and how it can be achieved in Chapter 18.

Exercise 11.2

(a) Explain briefly why, in Table 11.3, age and sex differences between the groups have to be adjusted for. (b) What do the results indicate about exercise as a risk factor for stroke among the 25–40 years and 40–55 years groups?

Exercise 11.3

Refer back to Table 1.3, the results from a cross-section study into thrombotic risk during pregnancy. Identify and interpret any statistically significant odds ratios.

VI

PUTTING IT TO THE TEST

12

TESTING HYPOTHESES ABOUT THE *DIFFERENCE* BETWEEN TWO POPULATION PARAMETERS

Learning objectives

When you have finished this chapter you should be able to:

- *Explain how a research question can be expressed in the form of a testable hypothesis*
- *Explain what a null hypothesis is*
- *Summarise the hypothesis test procedure*
- *Explain what a p-value is*
- *Use the p-value to appropriately reject or not reject the null hypothesis*
- *Summarise the principal tests described in this chapter, along with their most appropriate application, and any distributional and other requirements which must be satisfied*
- *Interpret SPSS and Minitab results from a hypothesis test*
- *Interpret published results of hypothesis tests*
- *Point out the advantages of confidence intervals over hypothesis tests*
- *Describe type I and type II errors, and their probabilities*
- *Explain what the power of a test measures, and how it is calculated*
- *Explain the connection between power and sample size*
- *Calculate sample size required in some common situations*

The Research Question and the Hypothesis Test

The procedures discussed in the preceding three chapters have one primary aim: to estimate, as precisely as possible, population parameter values. This approach enabled us to make statements like "We are 95% confident that the range of values defined by the confidence interval will include the value of the population parameter". Or, "The confidence interval represents a plausible range of values for the population parameter". There is, however, an alternative approach, that of *hypothesis testing*, which uses exactly the same sample data as does estimation, but focuses not on *estimating* a parameter value, but on *testing* whether a parameter has some specified value.

In recent years, the estimation approach has become more generally favoured, primarily because the results from a confident interval provides more information than the results of a hypothesis test (as you will see shortly). However, hypothesis testing is still popular in some situations, either because an appropriate computer program is not readily available, or because the more limited information produced by a hypothesis test is sufficient for the purpose and the test is easy to perform, or because alternative estimation procedures have not been developed or established. For these reasons I will describe a few of the more commonplace tests. Let's first of all establish some basic concepts.

THE NULL HYPOTHESIS

As you saw at the beginning of Chapter 6, almost all investigations begin with a question: "Does exercise earlier in life reduce the chances of experiencing a stroke later in life?", "Is a new drug for hypertension more effective than an existing drug of choice?", "Do bottle fed babies experience more sudden infant death syndrome (SIDS) than breast fed babies?", and so on. To answer questions like this you have to transform the research question into a *testable hypothesis* of the form:

Hypothesis: Exercise does NOT reduce stroke risk.

Hypothesis: The new drug is NOT more effective at reducing hypertension than the existing drug.

Hypothesis: Bottle-fed babies do NOT experience more, or less, SIDS than breast-fed babies.

Notice that all of these hypotheses reflect the conservative position of *no* change, *no* effect, *no* difference, etc., and for this reason are called *null* hypotheses. Usually researchers have reason to believe that there *is* some effect or some difference (that's often the prime reason for the research!), and they will take samples and measure outcomes in the hope of finding strong-enough evidence to be able to refute or *reject* the null hypothesis as not true.

The Process

The hypothesis testing process can be summarised thus:

- Use your research question to define an appropriate and testable null hypothesis.
- Select a suitable outcome variable.
- Collect the appropriate sample data and determine the relevant sample statistics.
- Define a rule which will enable you to judge whether the sample evidence is strong enough for you to reject the null hypothesis, or not.
- Examine the sample statistics for evidence against the null hypothesis, and make a judgement, depending on the strength of this evidence, either to reject or not reject the null hypothesis.

Let's take a simple example. Suppose you play a coin-tossing game—heads you win, tails you loose. Your opponent is the clinic practical joker, so before agreeing to play, you decide to toss the coin 100 times, and see how many heads and tails you get. Too few tails will be evidence of coin tampering, and you won't play. You assume that the coin is fair; i.e. your null hypothesis is that the coin is *not* biased. Now, even if the coin is fair you know that you're unlikely to get exactly 50 tails and 50 heads, because of the element of chance. So how small a number of tails (or heads) would you have to get before you suspect the coin to be fixed—45, 40, 30? Picking a number out of thin air is obviously not very satisfactory, and what you need is a general decision rule based in some way on the minimum number of tails you could *expect* to get if the coin was fair. This is your line in the sand. If the number of tails falls below this expected number, you will reject the null hypothesis that the coin is fair. How then are you to derive such a decision rule?

The *p*-value

Statisticians have devised the following convention: if the probability of getting the number of tails you do get (or even fewer) is *less than 0.05 or 0.01*,[1] when the null hypothesis is assumed to be true, then this is strong enough evidence against the null hypothesis to enable you to reject it. The beauty of this rule is that you can apply it to any situation where the probability of an outcome can be calculated, not just to coin tossing.

In your coin-tossing game you would have to work out how many tails (or fewer) would have a probability of only 0.05 of occurring if you tossed the coin 100 times. If the actual number of tails you get is less than this, you will reject the null hypothesis. Now the number of tails (or heads) in any given number of tosses of a coin follows the binomial distribution, and the probability of getting say 42 *or fewer* tails if the coin is fair turns out to be 0.0666, which is not less than 0.05 (Table 12.1). This is *not* strong enough evidence against the null hypothesis. However, the probability of getting *41 or fewer* tails is 0.0443, which *is* less than 0.05. This is strong enough evidence.

So your rule becomes: if you get *41 or fewer tails* in 100 tosses of the coin, you will reject the null hypothesis of a fair coin, and conclude that the coin is fixed. This outcome probability, 0.0443 in this example, is called the *p-value*, and is defined thus:

> A *p*-value is the probability of getting the output observed (or one more extreme), assuming the null hypothesis to be true.

So the decision rule in the end is simple:

- Determine the *p-value* for the output you have obtained (using a computer).
- Compare it with the *critical value*, usually 0.05, but sometimes 0.01.
- If the *p*-value is *less* than the critical value, reject the null hypothesis; otherwise do not reject it.

When you reject a null hypothesis, it's worth remembering that although there is a probability of 0.95 that you are making the correct decision, there is a

---

[1] There is nothing magical about these values, they are quite arbitrary.

Table 12.1 Percentage probability of getting between 30 *or fewer* tails, and 50 *or fewer* tails, in 100 tosses of a coin, assuming that the coin is fair; i.e. that the probability of a tail is 0.50. This was obtained from Minitab. Notice that for fewer than 30 tails, the probabilities are all shown as 0.0000. These probabilities are not zero, but are so small that four decimal places doesn't capture them

NO. OF TAILS	CUMULATIVE PROBABILITY (%)
30	0.0000
31	0.0001
32	0.0002
33	0.0004
34	0.0009
35	0.0018
36	0.0033
37	0.0060
38	0.0105
39	0.0176
40	0.0284
41	0.0443
42	0.0666
43	0.0967
44	0.1356
45	0.1841
46	0.2421
47	0.3086
48	0.3822
49	0.4602
50	0.5398

corresponding probability of 0.05 that your decision is incorrect. You can't be certain that your decision is correct, but there are 95 chances in 100 that it is. Compare this with the conclusion from a confidence interval where you can be 95% confident that a confidence interval will include the population parameter, but there's still a 5% chance that it will not.

It's important to stress that the *p*-value is *not* the probability that the null hypothesis is true (or not true); it's a measure of the *strength of the evidence against* the null hypothesis. The smaller the *p*-value, the stronger the evidence (the less likely the outcome occurred by chance). Note that the critical value, usually 0.05 or 0.01, is called the *significance level* of the hypothesis test and denoted α (alpha). We'll return to alpha again shortly.

So for any hypothesis test all you need to do is examine the associated *p*-value, observe whether it's less than 0.05, and decide accordingly. Calculating *p*-values by hand can be difficult, but most computer programs provide them.

Exercise 12.1

Suppose in the coin-tossing example you decided to set the significance level at (a) 0.1, and (b) 0.01. Use Table 12.1 to decide on the number of tails (or fewer) which would cause you to reject the null hypothesis of a fair coin in each case. (Assume probabilities of 30 tails or fewer are all actually zero.)

There are as you might expect numerous different hypothesis tests used in clinical work. Outside the specialist applications, the three most common applications are for tests to determine:

- whether a particular parameter in two populations are equal (i.e. the difference between them is zero)
- whether a particular parameter is the same size in two populations (i.e. their ratio is equal to 1)
- whether a particular parameter in two populations is distributed with equal proportions across a number of categories.

I'll discuss each of these situations in detail shortly.

Some hypothesis tests are suitable only for metric data, some for metric and ordinal data, and some for ordinal and nominal data. Some require data to have a particular distribution (often Normal)—these are *parametric* tests. Some have no distributional requirements—the *non-parametric* tests. I have listed below a brief summary of the more commonly used tests for two populations, along with their data and distributional requirements, if any. I am ignoring tests of single population parameters since these are not often enough required.

BRIEF SUMMARY OF A FEW OF THE COMMONEST TESTS

The two-sample *t*-test
Used to test whether or not the difference between two *independent* population means is zero (i.e. the two means are equal). The null assumption is that it is zero. Data must be metric, and both variables Normally distributed (this is a parametric test). In addition the two population standard deviations should not be too different (although for larger sample sizes this becomes less important).

The matched-pairs *t*-test
Used to test whether or not the difference between two *paired* population means is zero. The null assumption is that it is (i.e. the two means are equal). Data must be metric, and the *differences* between the two variables Normally distributed (this is a parametric test).

The Mann–Whitney test
Used to test whether or not the difference between two *independent* population medians is zero. The null assumption is that it is (i.e. the two medians are equal). Data must be either metric or ordinal. There is no requirement as to the actual distributional shape of the populations, but they are required to be similar. This is the non-parametric equivalent of the two-sample *t*-test.

The Wilcoxon test
Used to test whether or not the difference between two *paired* population medians is zero. The null assumption is that it is (i.e. the two medians are equal). Data must be either metric or ordinal. There is no requirement as to distributional shape, but

the *differences* should be distributed reasonably symmetrically. This is the non-parametric equivalent of the matched-pairs *t*-test.

The chi-squared test

Used to test whether the proportions across a number of categories of two or more *independent* groups is the same. The null hypothesis is that they are. Data may be categorical, ordinal, metric discrete (provided the number of categories is small), or metric continuous, if grouped into a small enough number of groups.[2] The chi-squared (χ^2) test is also a test of the independence of the two variables, and has a number of other applications (as you will see).

Fisher's exact test

Used to test whether the proportions in two categories of two *independent* groups is the same. The null hypothesis is that they are. Data may be categorical, ordinal, metric discrete (provided the number of categories is small), or metric continuous if grouped into a small enough number of groups. This test is an alternative to the chi-squared test in the two-category/two-group case (known as a 2×2), when the results from a chi-squared test indicate too little data in some cells (I'll explain this later).

McNemar's test

Used to test whether the proportions in two categories of two *matched* groups is the same. The null hypothesis is that they are. Data may be categorical, ordinal, metric discrete (provided the number of categories is small), or metric continuous, if grouped into a small enough number of groups.

The Two-sample t-test

Since the two-sample *t*-test is one of the more commonly used hypothesis tests, and we already have the relevant output, it will be helpful to see how to interpret the computer output. For example, let's apply the two-sample *t*-test to test the null hypothesis of no difference in the mean birthweights of maternity unit-born and home-born infants (data in Table 10.1).

With SPSS

Look back at Figure 10.1, which shows the output from SPPS, which in addition to the 95% confidence interval gives the result of the two-sample *t*-test of the equality of the two population mean birthweights. The test results are given in columns five, six and seven. The column headed "Sig. (2-tailed)" gives the *p*-value, 0.407. Since this is not less than 0.05 you cannot reject the null hypothesis, and you thus conclude that there is no difference in the two population mean birthweights.

With Minitab

The Minitab output in Figure 10.2 gives the same value as SPSS for the *p*-value of 0.407, shown in the bottom row, confirming that the two means are equal.

---

[2] What is a small enough number of categories depends largely on sample size, but five or six seems a practical maximum in most cases. With too many categories there is a danger that some cells will have very small numbers.

SOME EXAMPLES OF HYPOTHESIS TESTS FROM PRACTICE
Two Independent Means: The Two-sample *t*-test

Table 12.2 shows the baseline characteristics of two independent groups in a randomised controlled trial to compare conventional blood pressure measurement (CBP), and ambulatory blood pressure measurement (ABP), in the treatment of hypertension. *p*-Values for the differences in the basic characteristics of the two groups are shown in the last column.

Table 12.2 Baseline characteristics of two *independent* groups from a randomised controlled trial to compare conventional blood pressure measurement (CBP), and ambulatory blood pressure measurement (ABP), in the treatment of hypertension. *p*-Values of the differences in group parameter values are shown in the last column

CHARACTERISTICS	CBP GROUP (n = 206)	ABP GROUP (n = 213)	p
Age, mean (SD) (years)	51.3 (11.9)	53.8 (10.8)	0.03
Body mass index, mean (SD), kg/m^2	28.5 (4.8)	28.2 (4.4)	0.39
Women, no. (%)	102 (49.5)	124 (58.2)	0.07
Receiving oral contraceptives, no. (%)*	14 (13.7)	10 (8.1)	0.17
Receiving hormonal substitution, no. (%)*	19 (18.6)	19 (15.3)	0.51
Previous antihypertensive treatment, no (%)†	134 (65.0)	139 (65.3)	0.95
Diuretics, no. (%)*	47 (35.1)	59 (42.4)	0.26
β-blockers, no. (%)*	65 (48.5)	80 (57.6)	0.17
Calcium-channel blockers, no. (%)*	45 (33.6)	38 (27.3)	0.32
Angiotensin-converting enzyme inhibitors, no. (%)*	50 (37.3)	48 (34.5)	0.72
Multiple-drug treatment, no. (%)*	62 (46.3)	65 (46.8)	0.97
Smokers, no. (%)	42 (20.5)	35 (16.4)	0.29
Alcohol use, no. (%)	115 (55.8)	102 (47.9)	0.10
Serum creatinine, mean (SD), μmol/L‡	85.75 (15.91)	88.4 (16.80)	0.25
Serum total cholesterol, mean (SD), mmol/L‡	6.00 (1.03)	6.10 (1.19)	0.32

*Percentages and values of *p* computed considering only women receiving antihypertensive drug treatment before their enrollment.
†Defined as antihypertensive drug treatment within 6 months before the screening visit.
‡Divide creatinine by 88.4 and cholesterol by 0.02586 to convert to milligrams per decilitre.

The authors used a variety of tests to assess the difference between a number of different parameters for these independent groups (although these are referred to in the text, this information should have been available somewhere in the table itself). To assess the difference in population mean age and mean body mass index (BMI), they used a two-sample *t*-test. For age, the *p*-value is 0.03, so you can reject the null hypothesis of equal mean ages and conclude that the difference is statistically significant. The *p*-value for the difference in mean BMIs is 0.39, so you can conclude that the BMIs in the two populations are the same. Note that *differences in independent percentages* can also be tested with the two-sample *t*-test.

Exercise 12.2
Comment on what the results in Table 12.2 indicate about the difference between the two populations in terms of their mean serum creatinine and serum total cholesterol levels.

Exercise 12.3
Refer back to Table 1.2, showing the basic characteristics of women in the breast cancer and stressful life events case–control study. Comment on what the p-values tell you about the equality or otherwise, between cases and controls, of the means of the seven metric variables.

Two Matched Means: the Matched-pairs *t*-test

Table 10.3 provides an example from practice, and shows the p-values for the differences in population mean bone mineral densities between two individually matched groups of depressed and normal women (which we have already discussed in confidence-interval terms). As you can see, only at the radius is the population mean bone mineral density the same, with a p-value of 0.25. All the other p-values are less than 0.05. Notice that this confirms the confidence-interval results, also given. Note that differences in matched percentages can also be tested with the matched-pairs *t*-test.

Two Independent Medians: the Mann–Whitney Test

With ordinal data or metric data, for which the median is the preferred measure of location—perhaps because of skewed data—and with two independent groups, the Mann–Whitney test can be used to test the null hypotheses that the two population medians are the same. Recall that in Chapter 10, I introduced the Mann–Whitney procedure to calculate confidence intervals for the difference between two independent population median treatment times, from a randomised controlled trial into the use of ketorolac versus morphine to treat limb injury pain. Table 10.4 contains both 95% confidence intervals and p-values for a number of patient treatment times from this study.

You will recall that you found that only one confidence interval did not include 0, that for the time between receiving analgesia and leaving A&E (4.0 to 39.0), and this has a p-value of 0.02, less than 0.05. This confirms the fact that the difference in treatment time between the two population median times is statistically significant. However, there is a problem with the time for preparation of the analgesia. Table 10.4 shows this has a 95% confidence interval of (0 to 5.0), which includes 0, implying no significant difference in treatment times. But the p-value is given as 0.0002, which suggests a highly significant difference in population medians. In the accompanying text the authors indicate that this difference is significant, and quote the low p-value, so I can only assume a typographical error in the confidence interval.

Interpreting Computer Output for the Mann–Whitney Test

In view of the widespread use of the Mann–Whitney test, you might find it helpful to see the output for this procedure from SPSS and Minitab.

With SPSS
Using the Apgar scores in Table 10.1, you can use the Mann–Whitney to test whether the population median Apgar scores for infants born in a maternity unit and those born at home are the same. The null hypothesis is that the median Apgar scores are equal. The output from SPSS is shown in Figure 12.1, with a

p-value, labelled "Asymp. Sig. (2-tailed)", of 0.061. Since this is not less than 0.05 you cannot reject the null hypothesis of no difference in population median Apgar scores between the two groups, and you must conclude that they are the same.

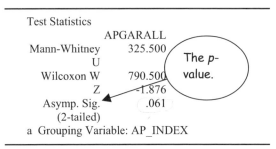

Test Statistics

	APGARALL
Mann-Whitney U	325.500
Wilcoxon W	790.500
Z	-1.876
Asymp. Sig. (2-tailed)	.061

a Grouping Variable: AP_INDEX

The p-value.

Figure 12.1: Output from SPSS for the Mann–Whitney test of the difference between medians of the two independent Apgar scores (raw data in Table 10.1)

With Minitab

Using the Apgar scores again, if you refer back to Figure 10.4, you will see the results of Minitab's Mann–Whitney test three rows from the bottom.[3] The *p*-value is given in the second row up as 0.0616, and since this is *not* less than 0.05 you *cannot* reject the null hypothesis. This is confirmed in the bottom row of the table, and enables you to conclude that the population median Apgar scores are the same in both groups of infants.

Two Matched Medians: the Wilcoxon test

In the same circumstances as for the Mann–Whitney test described above, but with individually matched pairs, the Wilcoxon test is appropriate. Look back at Table 10.5, which was from a matched case-control study into the dietary intake of schizophrenic patients living in the community in Scotland. Here the authors have used the Wilcoxon matched-pairs test for differences in the population median daily intakes of a number of substances between "All Patients" and "All Controls". The *p*-values are in the column headed "*p*", and as you can see the only *p*-value *not* less than 0.05 is that for protein (*p*-value = 0.07), so this is the only substance whose median daily intake does *not* differ between the two populations. Once again this confirms the confidence-interval results.

Confidence Intervals Versus Hypothesis Testing

I said at the beginning of this chapter that, where possible, confidence-interval estimation is preferred to hypothesis testing because the confidence intervals are more informative. How so?

Look back at Table 10.4 from the randomised controlled trial comparing ketorolac and morphine for limb injury pain. The authors give both 95% confidence intervals and *p*-values for differences in a number of different treatment times between

---

[3] ETA is Minitab's word for the population median.

two groups of limb injury patients. Let's take the last of these. For the "Interval between receiving analgesia and leaving A&E", the p-value of 0.02 would enable you to reject the null hypothesis and conclude that the difference between the two population median treatment times is statistically significant.

The 95% confidence interval of (4.0 to 39.0) minutes, tells us, not only that the difference between the population medians is statistically significant—because the confidence interval does not contain 0—but in addition, that the value of this difference in population medians is likely to be somewhere between 4.0 minutes and 39 minutes. So the confidence interval does everything that the hypothesis test does: it tells us whether the medians are equal or not, but it also gives us extra information—on the likely range of values for this difference. Moreover, unlike a p-value, the confidence interval is in clinically meaningful units, which helps with the interpretation. As a consequence you should if possible use confidence intervals in preference to p-values.

NOBODY'S PERFECT: TYPES OF ERROR

Suppose you are investigating a new drug for the treatment of hypertension. Your null hypothesis is that the drug has no effect. Now suppose the drug *does* actually reduce mean systolic blood pressure, but by only 5mmHg, but the hypothesis test you use can only detect changes of 10mmHg or more. As a consequence, you will not find strong enough evidence to reject the null hypothesis, and so you'll conclude, mistakenly, that the new drug is not effective. Of course, the effect is there, it's just that your test does not have enough *power* to detect it. You need to improve the power of the test so that it will detect differences as small as 5mmHg, but how? Before I address this question, first a few words on types of error.

So when you decide either to reject or not reject a null hypothesis on the evidence of a p-value, you could be making a mistake. After all you are basing your decision on sample (not population) evidence. Even if you have done everything right, your sample could still, by chance, not be very representative of the population, or it could simply be too small to pick up enough evidence. There are two possible errors:

- *Type I error*—rejecting a null hypothesis when it is true (also known as a *false positive*). In other words, you conclude there is an effect when there isn't. The probability of committing a type I error is denoted α (alpha), and is the same alpha as the significance level of a test.
- *Type II error*—not rejecting a null hypothesis when it is false (also known as a *false negative*). That is, you conclude there is no effect when there is. The probability of committing a type II error is denoted β (beta).

So when you set the significance level of a hypothesis test to $\alpha = 0.05$, it's because you want the probability of a type I error to be 0.05. Obviously you would like a test procedure which minimised this probability, because in many clinical situations a type I error is potentially serious—judging some procedure to be effective when it is not. Nonetheless, if there *is* a real effect you would certainly like to detect it, so you also want to minimise the probability of β, a type II error; or put another way, you want to make $(1 - \beta)$ as large as possible.

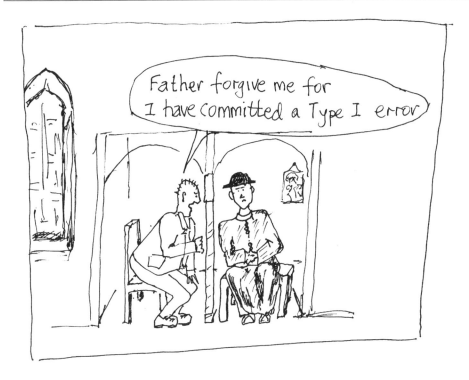

THE POWER OF A TEST

In fact, the *power* of a test is defined to be (1 – β), and is a measure of its capacity to reject the null hypothesis when it is false; in other words, to detect an effect if one is present. In practice, β is typically set at 0.2 or 0.1, giving power values of 0.80 (or 80%) and 0.90 (or 90%), respectively. This means that if there is an effect, the test has a probability of detecting it of 0.80 or 0.90. Although you would like to minimise both α and β, unfortunately they are, for a given sample size, linked. You can't make β smaller without making α larger, and vice versa. So, when you decide a value for α, you are also inevitably fixing the value of β. The only way to reduce both simultaneously is to increase the sample size.

An Example from Practice

The following is an extract from the randomised controlled trial of epidural analgesic in the prevention of stump and phantom pain after amputation, referred to in Table 5.3, in which the authors of the study outline their thinking on power:

> The natural history of phantom pain after amputation shows rates of about 70%, and in most patients the pain is not severe. Since epidural treatment is an invasive procedure, we decided that a clinically relevant treatment should reduce the incidence of phantom pain to less than 30% at week 1 and then at 3, 6, and 12 months after amputation. Before the start of the study, we estimated that a sample size of 27 patients per group would be required to detect a between-group difference of 40% in the rate of phantom pain (type I error rate 0.05; type II error rate 0.2; power = 0.8).

Exercise 12.4

(a) Explain, with the help of a few clinical examples, why you would normally want to minimise α, when testing a hypothesis. (b) Alpha is conventionally set to 0.05 or 0.01. Why, if you want to minimise it, don't you set it at 0.001 or 0.000001, or even 0?

SAMPLE SIZE

The size of a sample is determined both by the chosen level of alpha, usually 0.05 or 0.01, and the power required, either 80% or 90%.[4] The sample size calculation can be summarised thus:

- Decide on the minimum size of the *effect* that would be clinically useful or otherwise of interest.
- Decide the significance level α, usually 0.05 or 0.01.
- Decide the power required, usually 80% or 90%.
- Do the sample size calculation, using a nomograph,[5] or some appropriate software, or the rule of thumb described below.

Minitab has an easy-to-use sample size calculator for the most commonly used tests. Machin *et al.* (1987) is a comprehensive collection of sample size calculations for a large number of different test situations.

Sample Size Rules of Thumb[6]

Comparing the means of two groups (metric data)

The required sample size n is given by the following expression:

$$n = \frac{2 \times SD^2}{E^2} \times k$$

SD is the population standard deviation (assumed equal in both populations). This can be estimated using the sample standard deviations, if they are available from a pilot study, say. Otherwise the standard deviation will have to be guessed using whatever information is available. E is the minimum change in the mean which would be clinically useful or otherwise interesting. k is a magic number which depends on the power and significance levels required, and is obtained from Table 12.3.

Table 12.3   Table of magic numbers for sample size calculations

SIGNIFICANCE LEVEL (α)	POWER ($1 - \beta$)			
	70%	80%	90%	95%
0.05	6.2	7.8	10.5	13.0
0.01	9.6	11.7	14.9	17.8

---

[4] These same sample size calculations also apply if you are calculating confidence intervals. Samples which are too small produce wide confidence intervals, sometimes too wide to enable a real effect to be identified.

[5] A nomograph can be found in Altman (1991).

[6] I am indebted to Andy Vail for this material.

For example, suppose you propose to use a case–control study to examine the efficacy of a program of regular exercise in treating moderately hypertensive patients, as an alternative to your current drug of choice. The minimal difference in mean systolic blood pressures between the cases (given the exercise program), and the controls (given the existing drug), you think clinically worthwhile is 10mmHg. You will have to make an intelligent guess as to the standard deviation of systolic blood pressure (assumed the same in both groups—see above), but information on this, and many other measures, is likely to be available from reference sources, from the research literature, from colleagues, etc. Let's assume the systolic blood pressure standard deviation is 12mmHg. If the power required is 80% with a significance level of 0.05, then from Table 12.3, $k = 7.8$ and the sample size required per group is:

$$n = \frac{2 \times 12^2}{10^2} \times 7.8 = 22.5.$$

So you will need at least 23 subjects in each of the two groups (always round up to the next highest integer) to detect a change of 10mmHg.

Comparing the proportions in two groups (binary data)

The required sample size n is given by:

$$n = \frac{[P_a \times (1 - P_a)] + [P_b \times (1 - P_b)]}{(P_a - P_b)^2} \times k.$$

P_a is the proportion with treatment a, P_b is the proportion with treatment b, so ($P_a - P_b$) is the effect size. k is the magic number from Table 12.3.

For example, suppose the percentage of elderly patients with pressure sores in a large district hospital is currently around 40%, or 0.40. You want to test a new pressure-sore-reducing mattress, and you would like the percentage with pressure sores to decrease to at least 20%, or 0.20. So $P_a = 0.40$, and $(1 - P_a) = 0.60$; $P_b = 0.20$, and $(1 - P_b) = 0.80$; so $(P_a - P_b) = (0.40 - 0.20) = 0.20$. If the power required is 80% and the significance level $\alpha = 0.05$, then the required sample size per group is:

$$n = \frac{(0.40 \times 0.60) + (0.20 \times 0.80)}{0.20^2} \times 7.8 = 78.0.$$

Thus you would need at least 78 subjects in each group.

Exercise 12.5
In (a) the hypertension example, and (b) the pressure sore example, what sample sizes would be required if power and significance levels were respectively: (i) 90% and 0.05; (ii) 90% and 0.01; (iii) 80% and 0.01?

Exercise 12.6
Suppose you are proposing to use a randomised controlled trial to study the effectiveness of St John's Wort as an alternative to an existing drug for the treatment of mild to moderate depression. The percentage of patients reporting an improvement in mood 3 months after existing drug treatment is 70%. You would be satisfied if the percentage reporting mood improvement after 3 months' of St John's Wort was 80%. How big a sample would you require to detect this improvement if you wanted your test to have: (a) 80% power and an α of 0.05; (b) 90% power and an α of 0.01?

13

TESTING HYPOTHESES ABOUT THE *RATIO* OF TWO POPULATION PARAMETERS

> *Learning objectives*
>
> When you have finished this chapter you should be able to:
>
> - *Describe the usual form of null hypothesis in the context of testing the ratio of two population parameters, and point out the differences from tests of population differences*
> - *Interpret published results on tests of risk and odds ratios*

TESTING THE RISK RATIO

In Chapter 11 you saw that if the confidence interval for a risk ratio contains 1, then the population risk ratio is not statistically significant (i.e. significantly different from 1), which in turn means that the factor in question is not a statistically significant risk. You can also use the hypothesis test approach to find out whether any departure in the sample risk ratio from 1 is statistically significant or due to chance. The null hypothesis is that the population risk ratio equals 1. If the associated *p*-value is less than 0.05 (or 0.01), then the population risk ratio in question is statistically significant, and the risk factor in question is a significant risk.

An Example from Practice

Table 13.1 is from a randomised trial into the efficacy of long-term treatment with subcutaneous heparin in unstable coronary-artery disease, and shows the risk ratios, 95% confidence intervals, and *p*-values for a number of clinical outcomes, in two independent groups, one group given heparin, the other a placebo.

As you can see from the *p*-values in the last column, three out of the six risk ratios were statistically significant: death, myocardial infarction, or both, at 1 month (*p*-value = 0.048); death, myocardial infarction, or revascularisation, at 1 month (*p*-value = 0.001); and death, myocardial infarction, or revascularisation, at 3 months (*p*-value = 0.031). All three of these *p*-values are less than 0.05, the remaining three are all greater than 0.05. Notice that these results are confirmed by the corresponding 95% confidence intervals.

Table 13.1   Risk ratios, 95% confidence intervals, and *p*-values, from a randomised trial into the efficacy of long-term treatment with subcutaneous heparin in unstable coronary-artery disease, for a number of clinical outcomes, at 1 month, 3 months and 6 months, in two independent groups, one group given heparin, the other a placebo

VARIABLE	DALTEPARIN (n = 1129)	PLACEBO (n = 121)	RISK RATIO (95% CI)	p
1 month				
Death, MI, or both	70 (6.2%)	95 (8.4%)	0.73 (0.54–0.99)	0.048
Death, MI, or revascularisation	220 (19.5%)	288 (25.7%)	0.76 (0.55–0.89)	0.001
3 months				
Death, MI, or both	113 (10.0%)	126 (11.2%)	0.89 (0.70–1.13)	0.34
Death, MI, or revascularisation	328 (29.1%)	374 (33.4%)	0.87 (0.77–0.99)	0.031
6 months*				
Death, MI, or both	148 (13.3%)	145 (13.1%)	1.01 (0.82–1.25)	0.93
Death, MI, or revascularisation	428 (38.4%)	440 (39.9%)	0.96 (0.87–1.07)	0.50

MI, = myocardial infarction.
*Delteparin (n = 1115), placebo (n = 1103).

Exercise 13.1
Table 13.2 is from a double-blind randomised controlled trial to assess the efficacy of tenecteplase as a possible alternative to alteplase in the treatment of acute myocardial infarction. The figure contains the risk ratios (relative risks), for a number of in-hospital cardiac events and procedures, for patients receiving tenecteplase compared to those receiving alteplase. (As a background note: rapid infusion of alteplase, with aspirin and heparin, is the current gold standard for pharmacological reperfusion in acute myocardial infarction. Tenecteplase is a mutant of alteplase with fewer of the limitations of alteplase.)

Identify and comment on those cardiac events and procedures which patients on alteplase had a statistically significant higher risk of experiencing than those on tenecteplase. Note: the key to the cardiac procedures is given in the table footnote. The Killip scale is a classification system for heart failure in patients with acute myocardial infarction, and varies from I (least serious, no heart failure, 5% expected mortality) to IV (most serious, cardiogenic shock, 90% expected mortality).

TESTING THE ODDS RATIO

Here the null hypothesis is that the population odds ratio is not significantly different from 1, and any departure from this value is due to chance. In other words, in the population the risk factor in question does not significantly increase or decrease the odds for the condition or disease. Only if the *p*-value for the sample odds ratio is less than 0.05 can you reject the null hypothesis and conclude that the risk factor is statistically significant and does change the odds by a statistically significant amount.

An Example from Practice

Table 13.3 is from an unmatched case–control study into the effect of passive smoking as a risk factor for coronary heart disease (CHD), in Chinese women who had never

Table 13.2 Relative risk for a number of non-cerebral bleeding complications in patients receiving tenecteplase compared to those receiving alteplase, from a double-blind RCT to assess the efficacy of tenecteplase compared to alteplase in the treatment of acute myocardial infarction

COMPLICATION	FREQUENCY (%)		RELATIVE RISK (95% CI)	p
	Tenecteplase (n = 8461)	Alteplase (n = 8488)		
Reinfarction	4.1	3.8	1.078 (0.929–1.250)	0.325
Recurrent angina	19.4	19.5	0.995 (0.935–1.058)	0.877
Sustained hypotension	15.9	16.1	0.988 (0.921–1.058)	0.737
Cardiogenic shock	3.9	4.0	0.965 (0.832–1.119)	0.664
Major arrhythmias	20.5	21.2	0.968 (0.913–1.027)	0.281
Pericarditis	3.0	2.6	1.124 (0.941–1.343)	0.209
Invasive cardiac procedures PTCA	24.0	23.9	1.006 (0.953–1.061)	0.843
Stent placement	19.0	19.7	0.968 (0.910–1.029)	0.302
CABG	5.5	6.2	0.884 (0.783–0.999)	0.049
IABP	2.6	2.7	0.968 (0.805–1.163)	0.736
Killip class >I	6.1	7.0	0.991 (0.982–0.999)	0.026
Tamponade or cardiac rupture	0.6	0.7	0.816 (0.558–1.193)	0.332
Acute mitral regurgitation	0.6	0.7	0.886 (0.613–1.281)	0.571
Ventricular septum defect	0.3	0.3	0.817 (0.466–1.434)	0.568
Anaphylaxis	0.1	0.2	0.376 (0.147–0.961)	0.052
Pulmonary embolism	0.09	0.04	2.675 (0.710–10.080)	0.145

PTCA, Percutaneous transluminal coronary angioplasty; CABG, coronary-artery bypass graft; IABP, intra-aortic balloon pump.

smoked. The cases were patients with CHD, the controls women without CHD. The study looked at the both passive smoking at home from husbands who smoked, and at work from smoking co-workers. The null hypothesis was that the population odds ratio was equal to 1 in each case; i.e. that passive smoking has no effect on the odds for CHD. The figure contains the adjusted odds ratios for CHD for a number of risk factors, with 95% confidence intervals and p-values.

The adjusted odds ratio for CHD from passive smoking by the husband was 0.94, with a p-value of 0.60, so you *cannot* reject the null hypothesis. You conclude that passive smoking by husbands is not a statistically significant risk factor for CHD in wives. The same conclusions can be drawn for the odds ratio of 1.85 for passive smoking at work, p-value equals 0.12.

Table 13.3 Odds ratios, 95% confidence intervals and *p*-values from an unmatched case–control study into the effect of passive smoking as a risk factor for coronary heart disease. The cases were patients with coronary heart disease, the controls individuals without coronary heart disease

	ADJUSTED ODDS RATIO (95% confidence interval)*	*p*-VALUE
Final model (factors 1 to 7):		
1 Age (years)	1.13 (1.04 to 1.22)	0.003
2 History of hypertension	2.47 (1.14 to 5.36)	0.022
3 Type A personality	2.83 (1.31 to 6.37)	0.008
4 Total cholesterol (mg/dl)	1.02 (1.01 to 1.03)	0.0006
5 High density lipoprotein cholesterol (mg/dl)	0.94 (0.90 to 0.98)	0.003
6 Passive smoking from husband	1.24 (0.56 to 2.72)	0.60
7 Passive smoking at work	1.85 (0.86 to 4.00)	0.12
Other model (factors 1 to 5 and passive smoking at work)	1.95 (0.90 to 4.10)†	0.087
Other model (factors 1 to 5 and passive smoking from husband or at work, or both)	2.36 (1.01 to 5.55)†	0.049

*Adjusted for the other variables in the final model.
†Adjusted for the first five variables above; odds ratios for these variables in the other models were essentially the same as those shown above and are not shown.

Exercise 13.2
Identify those risk factors in Table 13.3 which are statistically significant for CHD in the population from whom this sample of women was drawn.

14

TESTING HYPOTHESES ABOUT THE *EQUALITY* OF POPULATION PROPORTIONS

Learning objectives

When you have finished this chapter you should be able to:

- *Describe the rationale underlying the chi-squared test*
- *Explain the difference between observed and expected values*
- *Calculate expected values and the test statistic*
- *Perform a chi-squared test*
- *Interpret SPSS and Minitab chi-squared test results*
- *Interpret published results of chi-squared tests*
- *Outline the procedure for the chi-squared test for the independence of two variables*
- *Outline the procedure for the chi-squared test for trend*

THE CHI-SQUARED TEST

Two hypothesis tests are very prominent in general clinical research. The first is the two-sample *t*-test (see Chapter 12), used to test the equality of two independent population means or percentages, when the data is metric. The second is the *chi-squared test*,[1] used to test the equality of population proportions in two or more independent groups across two or more categories. The data is categorical (or can be made so, by grouping for example).

An Example

To explain the idea of the chi-squared test, let's start with the "2×2" table in Table 14.1. The columns represent the two groups "Smokers" and "Non-smokers", for the mothers of the infants whose data is shown in Table 10.1. These two groups are *independent*. This is a requirement of the chi-squared test (if the two groups are matched, then *McNemar's test* becomes appropriate). The rows of the table represent the two categories of the variable *birthing place* (maternity unit or home birth).

---

[1] The test is called the chi-squared test because it uses the *chi-squared* distribution. This is similar in shape to the Normal distribution when samples are large.

Table 14.1 *Observed* values in the sample of mothers giving birth in maternity units and at home, who smoked during their pregnancy (raw data in Table 10.1)

PLACE OF BIRTH	SMOKED		TOTALS
	Group 1: Yes	*Group 2: No*	
Maternity unit	10	20	30
Home	6	24	30
Totals	16	44	60

We want to answer the following question: "Is the proportion of mothers who smoked during pregnancy the same in the category 'Maternity unit' as it is in the category 'Home'?" Or equivalently, is the *difference* between the two proportions 0? The null hypothesis is that the two population proportions *are* the same; i.e. the difference between them is 0.

You know that 10 out of the sample of 30 maternity-unit mothers (a proportion of 0.333), and 6 out of 30 home-birth mothers (a proportion of 0.200), had smoked. These sample proportions are definitely *not* the same, but this could be due to chance. Now if the null hypothesis *was* true, then you would *expect* these two sample proportions to be more or less equal. Since we've got 16 smokers in a total of 60 women, a proportion of $16/60 = 0.2667$, you would expect to find 0.2667 of the 30 in each category, which is $0.2667 \times 30 = 8$. So you'd expect about 8 smokers in each group, rather than the observed values of 10 and 6.

An easier way to calculate expected frequencies is to use the expression:

Expected value for any cell = total of the row the cell is in
$\times$ total of the column the cell is in
$\div$ the overall total.

For example, for the top left-hand cell, the row total is 30, the column total is 16, and the overall total is 60, so the expected value is $(30 \times 16)/60 = 8$. Since the row totals are both 30, this means that the other two cells must each have an expected value of 22. In other words, the two-by-two table you would *expect* to see if the null hypothesis were true is that shown in Table 14.2.

Table 14.2 *Expected* values in the sample of mothers giving birth in maternity units and at home who smoked during their pregnancy, assuming the null hypothesis of equal proportions is true (raw data in Table 10.1)

PLACE OF BIRTH	SMOKED		TOTALS
	Group 1: Yes	*Group 2: No*	
Maternity unit	8	22	30
Home	8	22	30
Totals	16	44	60

Exercise 14.1

Calculate the expected values for the contingency table of "Mother smoked" and "Apgar score < 7", shown in Table 2.6.

Are the observed and expected values close enough?

As you've seen, even if the null hypothesis is true, you wouldn't expect the difference between the observed and expected values to be *exactly* 0. But how far away from 0 does this difference have to be before you accept that the sample results are indicative of a true difference in the proportions in the population, rather than a chance occurance? You can use the chi-squared test to answer this question: if the *p*-value associated with the chi-squared test is less than 0.05 (or 0.01), you can reject the null hypothesis, and conclude that there is a statistically significant difference in the proportions in each category.

Categories and groups

The chi-square test can be used with more than two categories and/or two groups, but with small sample sizes the maximum number of cells is limited by the proviso that none of the *expected* values should be less than 1, and that 80% of expected values should be greater than 5.[2] There are two ways around the problem of low expected values: first, increase the sample size (usually impractical); second, amalgamate two or more rows or columns, if this can be done and still make sense.

Doing the calculations

Calculation of a chi-squared test is not difficult to do by hand if the number of categories is small, but you would need a table of chi-squared values. The procedure is as follows:

- Calculate the expected value E, for each cell in the table.
- For each cell calculate the value of $O - E$, where O is the observed cell value.
- Square each $(O - E)$ value.
- Divide each $(O - E)^2$ value by the E value for that cell.
- Sum all of the values in the previous step.
- Take the square-root of the result from the previous step. This result is called the *test statistic*.[3]

To reject the null hypothesis of equal proportions, the value of the test statistic must exceed the critical chi-squared value obtained from a chi-squared table. For example, for a significance level of $\alpha = 0.05$, the test statistic must *exceed*: 3.84 for 2 × 2 table; 5.99 for a 2 × 3 table; 7.81 for a 2 × 4 table; and 12.59 for a 3 × 4 table. In practice you will probably use a computer program to do the chi-squared test, in which case you can simply use the *p*-value to reject or not the null hypothesis of equal proportions across categories. Figures 14.1 and 14.2 for an example, show

---

[2] There is some dispute among statisticians about the validity of this condition. Some suggest that the chi-squared test still works well even with low expected frequencies. Perhaps it is better to err on the side of caution.

[3] For the mathematically minded, the test statistic $= \sqrt{\sum \dfrac{(O - E)^2}{E}}$

the outputs from application of the chi-squared test to the smoking mothers example for both SPSS and Minitab. The programs produce identical results, with a *p*-value of 0.243 (and a test statistic of 1.364). Since this is *not* less than 0.05, you *cannot* reject the null hypothesis of equal population proportions of smokers in each category.

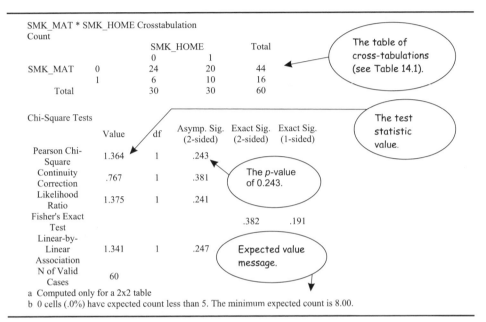

Figure 14.1: Output from the SPSS cross-tabs program with the chi-squared test option chosen, for the proportions of mothers who smoked during pregnancy among mothers giving birth in maternity units and at home

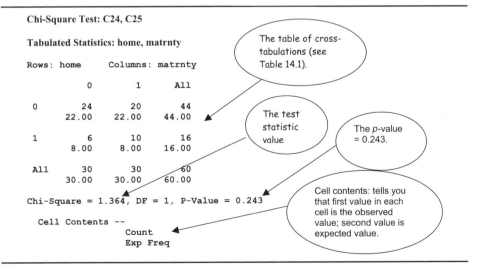

Figure 14.2: Output from the Minitab cross-tabs program with the chi-squared test option chosen, for the proportions of mothers who smoked during pregnancy among mothers giving birth in maternity units and at home

Exercise 14.2
Calculate the value of the test statistic using the expected values you calculated in Exercise 14.1. Can you reject the null hypothesis of equal proportions of smokers in both Apgar groups? Explain.

An Example from Practice

Table 14.3 is from the randomised controlled trial into ketorolac versus morphine for the treatment of limb pain (see Table 10.4), and shows the basic characteristics of the patients. The chi-squared test has here been used four times to test whether the proportions (expressed as percentages) in the ketorolac group and the morphine group are the same. First for the the proportion of men (categories "Men" and "Not men"); then for

Table 14.3   Basic characteristics of patients in the randomised controlled trial of ketorolac versus morphine for the treatment of blunt injury limb pain. Values are numbers (percentages*) unless stated otherwise

VARIABLE	KETOROLAC GROUP (n = 75)	MORPHINE GROUP (n = 73)	p-VALUE
Mean (SD) age (years)	53.9 (21.7)	53.2 (21.8)	0.85‡
No. (%) of men	38 (51)	33 (45)	0.51§
Mean (SD) body mass index (kg/m²)	22.8 (3.2)	23.0 (3.7)	0.77‡
Mean (interquartile range) time between injury and arrival at hospital (minutes)	95 (30–630)	82 (33–921)	0.75
Cause of injury:			
Motor vehicle crash	6 (8)	4 (5)	0.58¶
Falls	46 (61)	51 (70)	
Crush	20 (27)	14 (19)	
Other	3 (4)	4 (5)	
Fractures:	50 (67)	48 (66)	0.91§
Clavicle, humerus, elbow	5 (7)	8 (11)	
Radius, ulnar	8 (11)	11 (15)	
Hand	15 (20)	13 (18)	
Femur, patella	14 (19)	12 (16)	
Tibia, fibula	5 (7)	3 (4)	
Foot	2 (3)	1 (1)	
Non-fractures:			
Dislocation, upper limb	2 (3)	1 (1)	
Soft tissue injury, upper limb	10 (13)	10 (14)	
Soft tissue injury, lower limb	14 (19)	14 (19)	
Inital mean (SD) pain score:			
At rest	3.8 (1.1)	3.9 (1.1)	0.65‡
With activity	8.1 (1.2)	8.1 (1.2)	0.85‡
Referred for orthopaedic assessment	41 (55)	36 (49)	0.52§
Admitted to hospital†	38 (51)	29 (40)	0.18§
Admitted with adverse effects	0	3 (4)	

*Percentage may not sum to 100 because of rounding.
†Patients admitted to hospital (to orthopaedic or emergency observation ward).
‡t-test for unpaired means comparison.
§χ^2 test.
¶Fisher's exact test.

fracture site; then for referred for orthopaedic treatment; and finally for whether admitted to hospital.

The chi-squared test applied to the fracture sites data, for example, tests whether the proportions between the two groups is the same for all six sites, and gives rise to a 2 × 6 table. As you can see, the *p*-value is 0.91, which is not less than 0.05, so you can conclude that the null hypothesis of equal proportions cannot be rejected. In fact, the *p*-values for the chi-squared tests on each of the other three items are also all considerably greater than 0.05, indicating no difference between the two groups in any of them.

Notice that the authors have used Fisher's Exact test (see Chapter 12 for a brief description) to compare the equality of the proportions between the two groups for cause of injury. This is almost certainly because of low expected values in some cells.

USING CHI-SQUARED TO TEST WHETHER TWO VARIABLES ARE INDEPENDENT

Look at the hair colour data in Figure 3.1 which shows the numbers of boys and girls by hair colour. Two separate variables are involved here, sex (with two categories) and hair colour (with four categories). The two *groups*, boys and girls, are independent of each other. The chi-squared test for equality of proportions could be used as above to test whether the proportions of boys to girls was the same in each hair colour category. However, this test is at the same time a test of whether the two *variables*, sex and hair colour, are *independent*. How come?

The null hypothesis is that the two variables *are independent*, and if this is true, then there is absolutely no reason why the proportions of boys to girls should *not* be the same for each age category. So if the proportions are the *same*, this is taken as evidence that the two variables are *independent*. The alternative is that they are in some way associated. This means that for the chi-squared test of the fracture site in the ketorolac versus morphine example above, the population proportions of ketorolac patients for each of the six fracture sites was the same. This indicates that the two variables, drug group and fracture site, are independent (i.e. they are not associated). This is good news since this is what the randomisation process is designed to achieve.

Exercise 14.3
Following on from Exercise 14.2, are the variables, mother smoked during pregnancy and an Apgar score less than 7, independent or associated?

THE CHI-SQUARED TEST FOR TREND

The *chi-squared trend test* is another useful application of the chi-squared distribution, and is appropriate if the variable has categories which can be ordered (i.e. are ordinal, discrete metric, or grouped metric continuous). I can best explain this test with a real example.

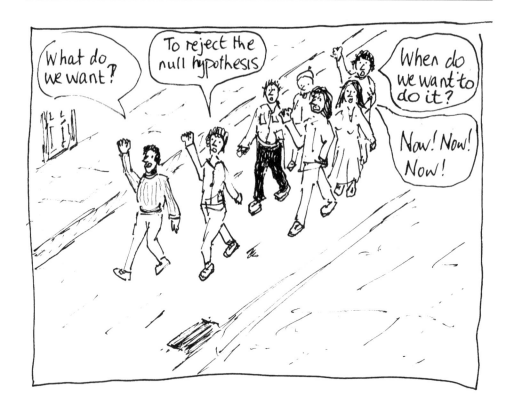

An Example from Practice

Look at Table 14.4, which shows the social class categories of the cases and controls in the unmatched case–control study of stressful life events as a potential risk factor for breast cancer in women (refer to Table 1.2). The subjects were women who attended with a breast lump. The cases were those women who received a malignant diagnosis, the controls those who received a benign diagnosis. These two groups are independent— since they are not matched.

Table 14.4 Numbers of subjects by social class among cases and controls in a study of stressful life events as a possible risk factor for breast cancer in women

SOCIAL CLASS	BREAST CANCER GROUP	NO BREAST CANCER CONTROL GROUP
I	10	20
II	38	82
III non-manual	28	72
III manual	13	24
IV	11	21
V	3	2
VI	3	4
Totals	106	226

With two groups and seven ordered categories of social class, we have a 2 × 7 table. If you apply the chi-squared test here, you are testing whether the proportion of breast cancer cases is the same in each social class category, and simultaneously whether the two variables, diagnosis and social class, are therefore independent. If the proportions are not the same you conclude that the variables are associated in some way.[4]

The problem is that if social class *is* associated with diagnosis, then you would *expect* the proportion getting a benign diagnosis to vary systematically, either increasing, or decreasing, as social class increased.[5] In other words, the variability in the proportions may be due largely to this trend, rather than to the fact that the variables are associated.

In the chi-squared test for trend, the null hypothesis is that there is *no* trend, and the *p*-value is used in the usual way. Notice that the test statistic for the trend test will always be less than that for the overall test described earlier. However, the trend test may produce a statistically significant result even when the overall test does not. This is because the test for trend is a more powerful test. The net result of all this is that, if one of your variables has ordinal categories, you should use the chi-squared test for trend rather than the overall chi-squared test.

As a matter of interest, the overall chi-squared test for the data in Table 14.4 gives a *p*-value of 0.784, while the chi-squared trend test gives a *p*-value of 0.094. As it happens, neither of these is statistically significant, but this is an illustration of how different the results from the two tests can be.

The chi-squared test has a large number of other applications, one of which we'll meet in Chapter 18.

Exercise 14.4
Refer back to Table 1.2, the breast cancer and stress case–control study. The table footnote indicates four chi-squared trend tests. Comment on what each *p*-value reveals about the existence of a trend in the categories of each of the variables concerned.

---

[4] Note that to perform the chi-squared test for trend we have to number the categories, for example, 1, 2, 3, etc.
[5] The direction of change would depend on whether stressful life events were more, or less, common in higher social class groups.

VII

GETTING UP CLOSE

15

MEASURING THE ASSOCIATION BETWEEN TWO VARIABLES

Learning objectives

When you have finished this chapter you should be able to:

- *Explain the meaning of association*
- *Draw and interpret a scatterplot, and from it assess the linearity, direction and strength of an association*
- *Distinguish between negative and positive association*
- *Explain what a correlation coefficient is*
- *Describe Pearson's correlation coefficient r, its distributional requirements, and interpret a given value of r*
- *Describe Spearman's correlation coefficient r_s, and interpret a given value of r_s*
- *Describe the circumstances under which Pearson's r or Spearman's r_s is appropriate*

ASSOCIATION

When we say that two variables are *associated*, we mean that they appear to behave in a way that makes them appear "interconnected"—changes in either variable seem to coincide with changes in the other variable. It's important to note (at this point anyway) that we are not suggesting that change in either variable is *causing* the change in the other variable, simply that they exhibit this connectedness.

In this chapter I want to discuss two alternative methods of detecting an association. The first method relies on a plot of the sample data, which can be ordinal or metric, using what is called a scatter diagram, scattergram, or *scatterplot*. A scatterplot will enable you to assess the existence and nature (strength and direction) of an association but only *qualitatively*, and thus has obvious limitations. For example, it's not always easy to say which of two sample scatterplots indicates the stronger association, and it doesn't allow us to make *inferences* about possible association in the population which was sampled.

The second approach is numeric, making both comparison and inference possible. I'll start with the qualitative, graphical approach, illustrated with some real examples.

THE SCATTERPLOT

As part of a cross-sectional study to examine the importance of parental smoking on passive exposure to tobacco smoke in schoolchildren, researchers calculated the cotinine concentrations in unexposed children (those children not exposed to smoking at home), randomly selected from 10 primary schools in 10 towns. Figure 15.1 is a scatterplot of cotinine concentrations in the unexposed children (as a percentage of their town mean), against the percentage of mothers who smoke in each town. It doesn't matter which variable is plotted on which axis for the scatterplot itself; but because the scatterplot is also important in the study of causal *relationships* between variables (which I will discuss in Chapter 17), it's a good idea to put what is called the *independent variable* on the horizontal axis, and the *dependent variable* on the vertical axis.

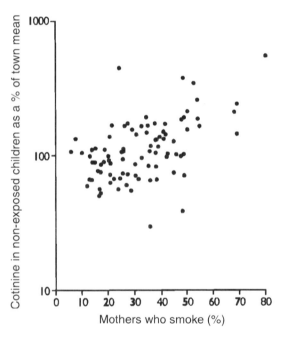

Figure 15.1: Scatterplot of cotinine levels in schoolchildren from 10 towns as a percentage of town means, and the percentage of mothers who smoke in each town, suggesting a positive association between the two variables

I'll have more to say about these terms later in the book, but for the moment you can ask yourself the question: "*If* there is a cause and effect relationship between the two variables, which variable is doing the causing and which is being affected as a consequence?" In this example, you would probably think that, if anything, smoking by mothers affects cotinine levels in children, rather than the other way round. So the variable being affected is cotinine level—this is the dependent variable and thus goes on the vertical axis. The variable acting on the cotinine level is the percentage of mothers who smoke, so this is the independent variable and is plotted on the horizontal axis. Incidentally, we usually talk about "plotting y against x"; that is, plotting the dependent variable against the independent variable, and not x against y.

From the scatterplot it's not difficult to see that something is going on here. The scatter is not just a completely random cloud of points, but appears to display a pattern—low cotinine levels seem to be associated with low percentages of mothers who smoke, and higher levels with higher percentages. You could justly claim that the two variables appear to be *positively associated*.

As a second example, Figure 15.2 shows a scatterplot taken from a study into the possible relationship between percentage mortality from aortic aneurysm, and the number of aortic aneurysm episodes dealt with per year, in each of 22 hospitals. This scatterplot displays a *negative association* between the two variables, because *low* values for number of episodes seem to be associated with *high* values for percentage mortality, and vice versa.

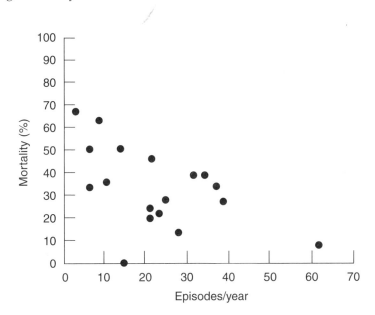

Figure 15.2: Scatterplot taken from a study into the possible relationship between percentage mortality from aortic aneurysm and number of aortic aneurysm episodes dealt with per year, in 22 hospitals, suggesting a negative association between the two variables

As a final example, Figure 15.3 shows a scatterplot taken from the cross-section study into the possible contribution of channel blockers (prescribed for depression) to the suicide rate in 284 Swedish municipalities, first referred to in Figure 3.11. The scatterplot here is very much more fuzzy than the two previous plots, and it would be hard to claim, merely from eyeballing it, that there is any significant association between the two variables (although admittedly there is some suggestion of a rather weak positive association).

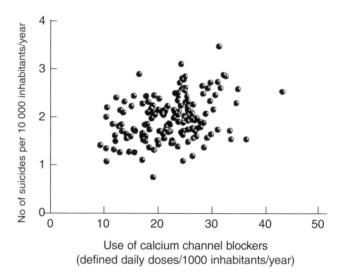

Figure 15.3: Scatterplot taken from a cross-section study into the possible contribution of channel blockers (prescribed for depression) and suicide rate in 152 Swedish munici-palities, suggesting a weak, if any, relationship between the variables

When you set out to investigate a possible association between two variables, a scatterplot is almost always worthwhile, and will often produce an insight into the way the two variables co-behave. In particular it may reveal whether an association between them is *linear*. The property of linearity is important in some branches of statistics, and we'll meet it again ourselves in Chapter 17. Put simply, a linear association is one in which the points in the scatterplot seem to cluster around a straight line. The two scatterplots in Figure 15.4 illustrate the difference between a linear and a non-linear association: the scatter on the left seems to be linear, but the one on the right shows some curviness.

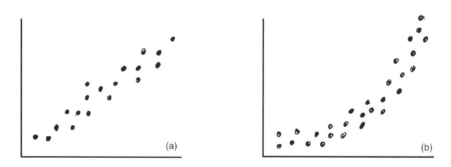

Figure 15.4: A linear association and a non-linear association

Exercise 15.1
Draw a scatterplot of Apgar score against birthweight for the 30 maternity-unit-born infants using the data in Table 2.1, and comment on what it shows about any association between the two variables.

Exercise 15.2

Cytomegalovirus (CMV) is a major problem for transplant patients. Researchers used a cohort study to identify early markers to predict patients at risk of CMV. They were exploring the possibility of using CMV load in the initial phase of active infection, along with the rate of increase of the viral load, as identifiers of patients at imminent risk of CMV disease. The scatterplot in Figure 15.5 shows peak viral load (log_{10}genomes/mL), plotted against initial viral load (log_{10}genomes/mL), in three different groups of transplant patients. In addition, the "best" straight line has been drawn through the points.[1] Comment on what the scatterplot suggests about the nature and strength of any association between the two variables.

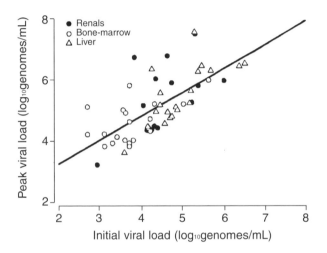

Figure 15.5: Scatterplot of peak viral load (log_{10}genomes/mL), against initial viral load (log_{10}genomes/mL), in three different groups of transplant patients, from a cohort study to identify early markers to predict patients at risk of CMV

Exercise 15.3

The scatterplot of percentage body fat against body mass index in Figure 15.6 is from a cross-section study into the relationship between body mass index (BMI) and body fat, in black populations in Nigeria, Jamaica and the USA. The aim of the study was to investigate whether percentage body fat rather than BMI could be used as a measure of obesity. What does the scatterplot tell you about the nature and strength of any association between these two variables?

THE CORRELATION COEFFICIENT

The principal limitation of the scatterplot in assessing association is that it does not provide us with a *numeric* measure of the strength of the association, but this is just what a *correlation coefficient* provides. Two correlation coefficients are widely used, Pearson's and Spearman's.

---

[1] I'll have more to say about what constitutes the best straight line in the next chapter. Loosely speaking, it's the line which passes as close as possible to all the points.

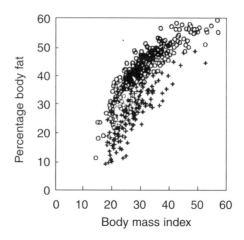

Figure 15.6: Scatterplot of percentage body fat against body mass index, from a cross-section study into the relationship between body mass index (BMI) and body fat, in black population samples from Nigeria, Jamaica and the USA

Pearson's Correlation Coefficient

Pearson's product–moment correlation coefficient, denoted ρ (Greek rho) in the population and r in the sample, measures the strength of the straight-line (i.e. linear) association between two variables. Both variables must be *metric continuous*, and approximately Normally distributed. The value of Pearson's r can vary from –1, indicating a perfect negative association (all the points exactly on the straight line); through 0, indicating no association; to +1, indicating perfect positive association (all points exactly on the line). Of course, in the real world, values of –1, 0 or +1 are never seen.

Loosely speaking, r is a measure of the *average* distance of all of the points from the "best" straight line that can be drawn through the scatter (this is analogous to the standard deviation measuring the average distance of each value from the mean).

Is the correlation coefficient statistically significant in the population?
To assess the statistical significance of a *population* correlation coefficient, you can use either the p-value (is it <0.05?), or the confidence intervals (does it include 0?). The null hypothesis is that the population correlation coefficient ρ is 0; i.e. there is no association. For example, for the data shown in the scatterplot in Figure 15.1, the sample r is 0.69 with a p-value of 0.02, indicating a statistically significant positive association between the two variables in the population. A useful rule of thumb, if you have a value for r but no confidence interval or p-value, is that to be statistically significant r must be greater than $2/\sqrt{n}$, where n is the sample size. For example, if n = 100, then r has to be greater than $2/10 = 0.200$, to be statistically significant.

An Example from Practice

Table 15.1 is taken from the same cross-section study into the relationship between body mass index (BMI) and body fat as Exercise 15.3, and shows the sample Pearson's correlation coefficient for the association of BMI and of percentage body fat, with blood pressure, and waist and hip measurements, along with an indication of the statistical significance or otherwise of the p-value.

Table 15.1 Correlation coefficients of body mass index (BMI) and body fat with waist and hip circumference, and blood pressure, in black population samples from Nigeria, Jamaica and the USA. The aim of the study was to investigate whether body fat rather than BMI could be used as a measure of obesity

VARIABLE	WOMEN						MEN					
	Nigeria		Jamaica		United States		Nigeria		Jamaica		United States	
	BMI	% fat	BMI	% fat	BMI	% fat	BMI	% fat	BMI	% fat	BMI	% fat
Waist circumference	0.90**	0.77**	0.87**	0.77**	0.91**	0.85**	0.89**	0.79**	0.69**	0.76**	0.93**	0.83**
Hip circumference	0.93**	0.81**	0.91**	0.82	0.93**	0.87**	0.89**	0.76**	0.64**	0.72**	0.93**	0.83**
Systolic blood pressure	0.24	0.24	0.16	0.15	0.21	0.21	0.09	0.09	0.24	0.24	0.24*	0.23*
Diastolic blood pressure	0.16	0.14	0.20	0.16	0.07	0.10	0.31	0.24	0.16	0.11	0.22	0.20

* $p < 0.05$; ** $p < 0.01$.

Unfortunately, the authors have not given the actual p-values but only indicated whether they were less than 0.05 or less than 0.01. This is not good practice: the actual p-values should always be provided. As you can see, the population correlation coefficient of both BMI and percentage body fat, with waist and hip circumference, is positive and statistically significant in every case. However, BMI is more *closely* associated (higher r values) than body fat, except in Jamaican men. Apart from the association with systolic blood pressure in US males, there is no statistically significant association with either of the blood pressure measurements.

Exercise 15.4
What would you guess the value of r is in Figure 15.5?

Exercise 15.5
Table 15.2 is from a case–control study of medical record validation, and shows the value of Pearson's r and the 95% confidence interval, for the correlation between gestational age, as estimated by the mother, and as determined from medical records, for a number of demographic sub-groups (ignore the last column). The cases were the mothers of child leukaemia patients, the matched controls were randomly selected by random telephone calling. Identify (a) any correlation coefficients not statistically significant, (b) the strongest correlation, (c) the weakest correlation.

Spearman's Rank Correlation Coefficient

If either (or both) of the variables is ordinal or not Normally distributed, then *Spearman's rank correlation coefficient* (r_s) is appropriate. This is a non-parametric measure, and it has the same value as Pearson's correlation coefficient when the latter is applied to metric data that has first been *ranked*. Spearman's r_s varies from -1 to $+1$, and its statistical significance can again be assessed with a p-value or a confidence interval. The null hypothesis is that the population correlation coefficient ρ_s is 0.

Table 15.2 Pearson's r_s and 95% confidence intervals, for the association between gestational age, as estimated by the mother, and from medical records, for a number of demographic subgroups, from a matched case–control study

	CORRELATION OF GESTATIONAL AGE	98% CI*	KAPPA STATISTIC†
All gestational ages	0.839	0.817–0.859	0.62
Case/control status			
Cases	0.849	0.813–0.878	0.63
Controls	0.835	0.805–0.861	0.61
Education			
<High school	0.694	0.553–0.797	0.51
Hight school	0.833	0.790–0.868	0.63
>High school	0.835	0.804–0.861	0.62
Household income			
<$22,000	0.791	0.734–0.837	0.59
$22,000–$34,999	0.882	0.849–0.908	0.62
≥$35,000	0.843	0.800–0.877	0.65
Unknown	0.745	0.641–0.823	0.60
Time (years) from delivery to interview			
<2	0.896	0.862–0.921	0.64
2–3.9	0.821	0.784–0.852	0.63
4–5.9	0.828	0.755–0.869	0.61
6–8	0.852	0.734–0.920	0.42
Maternal age (years)			
<25	0.822	0.773–0.861	0.64
25–29	0.889	0.862–0.912	0.63
30–34	0.760	0.694–0.813	0.57
≥35	0.888	0.824–0.930	0.64
Birth order			
First born	0.880	0.853–0.903	0.67
Second born	0.815	0.778–0.846	0.57
≥Third born	0.632	0.416–0.781	0.52
Maternal race			
White	0.846	0.822–0.866	0.64
Other	0.782	0.680–0.855	0.42

* CI, confidence interval.
† Three categories, <38, 38–41, ≥42 weeks.

An Example from Practice

Table 15.3 is from the same cross-section study first referred to in Figure 4.1, where variation in the use of the mammography services by 13,000 Canadian women (number of visits per 1000 women) was examined in relation to age group, across 33 district health councils. The authors wanted to know whether the variation in the ranked utilisation rates of the mammography service across the health districts was similar across the age groups. They proposed to do this by measuring the strength of the association between the ranked rates for each pair of different age groups. When the association was strong and significant they concluded that the variation in the usage rate was similar.

Table 15.3 Spearman correlation coefficients from a cross-section study of 13,000 Canadian women to examine the variation in the use of mammography services in relation to age group across 33 district health councils in Canada. Each correlation coefficient measures the strength of the association in the variation between the ranked usage rate across the health districts for each pair of age groups

AGE GROUP	30–39	40–49	50–69	70+
30–39	1.0000	0.6496 (p<0.0001)	0.5949 (p = 0.0005)	0.5488 (p = 0.0014)
40–49		1.0000	0.9021 (p<0.0001)	0.8985 (p<0.0001)
50–69			1.0000	0.9513 (p<0.0001)
70+				1.0000

The results show that the r_s for the association between the ranked usage rates for 30–39 year olds and 40–49 year olds across the 33 districts was 0.6496 (first row of the table), with a p-value of 0.0005. So this association is positive and statistically significant in these two age-group populations. Indeed, the correlation coefficients between all pairs of age groups is statistically significant, with all p-values less than 0.05. The authors thus concluded that variation in usage rate was similar for the four age groups across the 33 health districts. Whether association is the correct way to measure similarity in two sets of values is a question I will return to in the next chapter.

Exercise 15.6

Table 15.4 is from a study to develop and validate an outcome measure for palliative care. The Palliative-care Outcome Scale (POS) is designed for patients with advanced cancer and their families, and covers more than physical symptoms or quality-of-life related questions. The figure contains Spearman's r_s values for two associations, that between scores on the European Organisation for Research on Cancer Treatment Quality of Life Questionnaire (EORCT QLQ) and the patient-completed POS, and that between scores on the Support Team Assessment Schedule (STAS) and on the staff-completed POS. Each association was calculated for three items: physical symptoms, all non-quality-of-life problems, and quality of life. Comment on the results.

Table 15.4 Spearman's r_s values for two associations, that between scores on the European Organisation for Research on Cancer Treatment Quality of Life Questionnaire scale (EORCT QLQ), and the patient-completed Palliative-care Outcome Scale (POS), and that between scores on the Support Team Assessment Schedule (STAS), and on the staff-completed POS

SUBSCALE	EORCT QLQ–C30 v PATIENT POS (n = 29) (95% CI)		STAS v STAFF POS (n = 43) (95% CI)	
	Spearman's rho	p-value	Spearman's rho	p-value
Physical symptoms	0.51 (0.18 to 0.74)	0.005	0.80 (0.66 to 0.89)	0.000
All non-quality of life problems	0.53 (0.20 to 0.75)	0.003	0.67 (0.46 to 0.81)	0.000
Quality of life	0.43 (0.08 to 0.69)	0.022	0.51 (0.25 to 0.70)	0.001

Two other correlation coefficients can be mentioned only briefly. *Kendal's rank-order correlation coefficient*, denoted τ (tau), is appropriate in the same circumstances as Spearman's r_s—i.e. with ranked data (which may be ordinal or continuous). Tau is available in SPSS, but not in Minitab.

The *point-biserial* correlation coefficient is appropriate if one variable is metric continuous and the other is truly *dichotomous* (the variable can take only two values, alive or dead, male or female, etc.). Unfortunately, this latter measure of association is not available in either SPSS or Minitab.

AND FINALLY

If you plan to use a correlation coefficient you should ensure that the assumptions referred to in this chapter are satisfied, in particular that the association is linear—which you should always check with a scatterplot. Moreover, with Pearson's correlation coefficient you should interpret any results with suspicion if there are outliers present in either data set, since these can distort the results. Finally it is worth noting again that two variables being significantly associated does *not* mean that there is a cause-and-effect *relationship* between them.

16

MEASURING THE AGREEMENT BETWEEN TWO VARIABLES

Learning objectives

When you have finished this chapter you should be able to:

■ Explain the difference between association and agreement
■ Describe Cohen's kappa, calculate its value, and assess the level of agreement
■ Interpret published values for kappa
■ Describe the idea behind ordinal kappa
■ Outline the Bland–Altman approach to measuring agreement between metric variables

---

To Agree or Not Agree, That Is the Question

Association is a measure of the inter-connectedness of two variables, the degree to which they tend to change together, either positively or negatively. *Agreement* is the degree to which the values in two data sets actually *agree*. To illustrate this idea, look at the hypothetical data in Table 16.1, which shows the decision by a psychiatrist and a psychiatric social worker (PSW), whether to section (Y) or not section (N) each of 10 individuals with apparent mental ill-health. We would say that the two variables were in perfect agreement if every pair of values were the same. In practical situations this won't happen, and here you can see that only seven out of the 10 decisions are the same, so the *observed* level of *proportional agreement* is 0.70 (70%).

Table 16.1 Decision by a psychiatrist and a psychiatric social worker (PSW) whether or not to section 10 individuals suffering apparent mental ill-health

	PATIENT NUMBER									
	1	2	3	4	5	6	7	8	9	10
Psychiatrist	Y	Y	N	Y	N	N	N	Y	Y	Y
PSW	Y	N	N	Y	N	N	Y	Y	Y	N

COHEN'S KAPPA

But there is a problem. If you had asked each clinician simply to toss a coin to make the decision (heads—section, tails—don't section), some of their decisions would probably still have been the same, *by chance alone*. You need to adjust the observed level of agreement for the proportion you would have expected to occur anyway by chance alone. This adjustment gives us the *chance-corrected proportional agreement statistic*, Cohen's *kappa* (κ). So:

$$\kappa = \frac{\text{Proportion of observed agreement} - \text{Proportion of expected agreement}}{1 - \text{Proportion of expected agreement}}.$$

The expected proportions can be calculated from a 2×2 contingency table (just as with chi-squared), with the psychiatrist's scores in the rows, the PSW's scores in the columns, or vice versa. Table 16.2 shows this.

Table 16.2 Contingency table showing observed (and *expected*) decisions by a psychiatrist and a psychiatric social worker on whether to section 10 patients (data from Table 16.1)

PSYCHIATRIST	PSYCHIATRIC SOCIAL WORKER	
	Yes	*No*
Yes	4 (3)	2 (3)
No	1 (2)	3 (2)

We have seen that the observed agreement is 0.70, and we can calculate the expected agreement to be 5 out of 10, or 0.50. Therefore:

$\kappa = (0.70 - 0.50)/(1 - 0.50) = 0.20/0.50 = 0.40.$

So, after allowing for chance agreements, agreement is reduced from 0.70 or 70%, to 0.40 or 40%. Kappa can vary between 0 (agreement no better than chance) and 1 (perfect agreement), and you can use Table 16.3 to assess the quality of agreement. It's possible to calculate a confidence interval for kappa, but it will usually be too narrow (except for quite small samples) to add much insight.

Table 16.3 How good is the agreement?

KAPPA	STRENGTH OF AGREEMENT
<0.20	Poor
0.21–0.40	Fair
0.41–0.60	Moderate
0.61–0.80	Good
0.81–1.00	Very good

An Example from Practice

Table 16.4 is from the same Palliative-care Outcome Scale (POS) study as Table 15.3, and shows agreement between the patient and staff (who also completed the scale questionnaires) for a number of items on the POS scale. The table also contains values of Spearman's r_s, and the proportion of agreements within one point on the POS scale. The level of agreement between staff and patient is either fair or moderate for all items, and agreement within one point is either good or very good.

Table 16.4 From the same Palliative-care Outcome Scale (POS) study as Table 15.3, showing levels of agreement between the patients' and staff assessment for a number items on the POS scale. The figure also contains values of Spearman's r_s, and the proportion of agreements within one point on the POS scale?

ITEM	NO. OF PATIENTS	PATIENT SCORE (% severe)	STAFF SCORE (% severe)	κ (weighted)	SPEARMAN CORRELATION	PROPORTION AGREEMENT WITHIN 1 SCORE
At first assessment: 145 matched assessments						
Pain	140	24.3	20.0	0.56	0.67	0.87
Other symptoms	140	27.2	26.4	0.43	0.60	0.86
Patient anxiety	140	23.6	30.0	0.37	0.56	0.83
Family anxiety	137	49.6	46.0	0.28	0.37	0.72
Information	135	12.6	13.4	0.39	0.36	0.79
Support	135	10.4	14.1	0.22	0.32	0.79
Life worthwhile	133	13.6	16.5	0.43	0.54	0.82
Self worth	132	15.9	23.5	0.37	0.53	0.82
Wasted time	135	5.9	6.7	0.33	0.32	0.95
Personal affairs	129	7.8	13.2	0.42	0.49	0.96

Exercise 16.1
Do the highest and lowest levels of agreement in Table 16.4 coincide with the highest and lowest levels of correlation? Will this always be the case?

Exercise 16.2
Table 16.5 is from a study in a major trauma unit into the variation between two experienced trauma clinicians in assessing the degree of injury of 16 patients from their case notes, and shows the Injury Severity Scale (ISS) score awarded to each patient.[1] Categorise the scores into two groups: ISS scores of less than 16; and of 16 or more. Express the results in a contingency table, and calculate (a) the observed and expected proportional agreement, and (b) kappa. Comment on the level of agreement.

Table 16.5 ISS scores given by two experienced trauma clinicians to 16 patients in a major trauma unit

OBSERVER NO.	CASE NO.															
	1	2	3	4	5	6	7	8	9	10	11	12	13	14	15	16
1	9	14	29	17	34	17	38	13	29	4	29	25	4	16	25	45
2	9	13	29	17	22	14	45	10	29	4	25	34	9	25	8	50

---

[1] The ISS is widely used for the assessment of severity of injury, with a range from 0 to 75. ISS scores of 16 or above indicate potentially life-threatening injury, and survival with ISS scores above 51 is considered unlikely.

A limitation of kappa is that it is sensitive to the proportion of subjects in each category (i.e. to prevalence), so caution is needed when comparing kappa values from different studies—these are only helpful if prevalences are similar. Moreover, Cohen's kappa as described above is only appropriate for *nominal* data, as in the sectioning example above, although most data can be "nominalised", like the ISS values above. However, a version of kappa exists which can handle ordinal data.

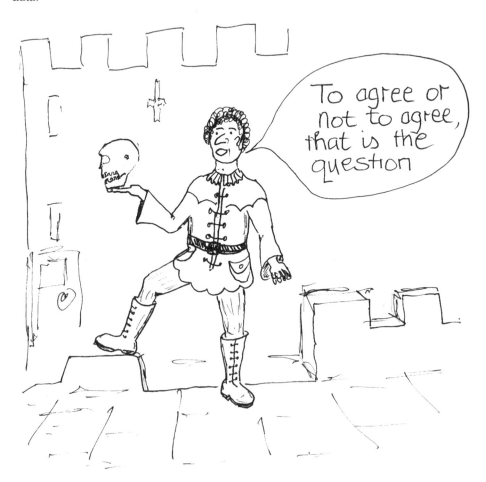

MEASURING AGREEMENT WITH ORDINAL DATA: WEIGHTED KAPPA

The idea behind weighted kappa is best illustrated by referring back to the data in Table 16.5. The two clinician's ISS scores agree for only five patients, so the proportional observed agreement is only 5/16 = 0.3125 (31.25%). But in several cases the scores have a "near miss": patient 2 for example, with scores of 14 and 13. Other pairs of scores are further apart: patient 15 is given scores of 25 and 8! Weighted kappa gives credit for near misses, but its calculation is too complex for this book.

MEASURING AGREEMENT BETWEEN TWO METRIC CONTINUOUS VARIABLES

The obvious problem with metric continuous data is the large number of possible values. It's quite possible that *none* of them will agree, and a cross-tabulation table is likely to have a large number of empty cells.

One solution is the Bland–Altman chart, which involves plotting, for each pair of measurements, the *differences* between the two scores on the vertical axis, against the *mean* of the two scores on the horizontal axis. A pair of tramlines, called the 95% *limits of agreement*, are drawn $\pm 2s_d$ (where s_d is standard deviation of the differences) each side of the zero difference line. If all the points on the graph fall between the tramlines, then agreement is "acceptable"; the more points there are outside the tramlines, the less good the agreement. Moreover, the spread of the points should be reasonably horizontal, indicating that differences are not increasing (or decreasing) as the values of the two variables increases.

An Example from Practice

The idea is illustrated in Figure 16.1, for agreement between diastolic blood pressure measured by patients at home with a cuff-measuring device (HP), and as measured by the same patients using an ambulatory device (ABPM). In this example there are only a few points outside the ±2 standard deviation tramlines and the spread of points is broadly horizontal.

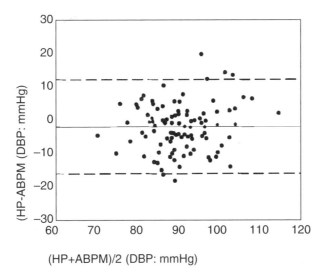

Figure 16.1: A Bland–Altman chart to measure agreement between two metric continuous variables, diastolic blood pressure as measured by patients at home with a cuff-measuring device (HP), and as measured by patients using an ambulatory device (ABPM)

To sum up, two variables that are in reasonable agreement will be strongly associated, but the opposite is not necessarily true. The two measures are not equivalent. *Association does not measure agreement.*

VIII

GETTING INTO A RELATIONSHIP

17

STRAIGHT-LINE MODELS: LINEAR REGRESSION

Learning objectives

When you have finished this chapter you should be able to:

- *Describe the difference between an association and a cause-and-effect relationship*
- *Estimate the equation of a straight line from a graph, and draw a straight line knowing the values of the constant and slope coefficients*
- *Describe what is meant by a linear relationship, and how the linear regression equation can be used to model it*
- *Identify the constant and slope parameters, and the dependent and independent variables*
- *Explain the role of the residual term*
- *Summarise the model-building process*
- *Provide a brief explanation of the idea behind the method of ordinary least squares estimation*
- *List the basic assumptions of the simple linear regression method*
- *Interpret computer-generated linear regression results*
- *Explain what goodness of fit is and how it is measured in the simple linear regression model*
- *Explain the role of $\bar{R}^2$ in the context of multiple linear regression*
- *Interpret published linear regression results*
- *Explain the adjustment properties of the regression model*
- *Outline how the basic assumptions can be checked graphically*

Health Warning!

Although the maths underlying the linear regression model is complicated, some explanation of the idea is necessary if you are to gain any understanding of the procedure, and be able to interpret regression computer outputs sensibly. I have tried to keep the discussion as brief and as non-technical as possible, but if you have an aversion to maths you might want to skim the material in the next few pages.

In Chapter 15, I emphasised the fact that an association between two variables does not mean that there is a cause-and-effect *relationship* between them. In the clinical world demonstrating a cause–effect relationship is difficult, and requires a number of conditions to be satisfied; for example, the relationship should be plausible, repeatable, predictable, with a proved mechanism, and them some. I will assume from here-on-in that a cause–effect relationship has been satisfactorily demonstrated. I want to start with a review of some school maths.

THE EQUATION OF A STRAIGHT LINE

Suppose you have the values shown below for two variables x and y, which when plotted result in a straight line (Figure 17.1):

y	2	3	4	6	7
x	0	2	4	8	10

You may remember that the equation of a straight line is $y = mx + c$, which I want to rewrite as:

$$y = b_0 + b_1 x.$$

The term b_0 is known as the *constant coefficient*, or the coefficient of intersection— it's where the line cuts the y axis. The term b_1 is known as the *slope coefficient*. This is positive if the line slopes upwards from left to right. (as in Figure 17.1), and negative if the line slopes down from left to right. Higher values of b_1 mean more steeply sloped lines. You can see from Figure 17.1 that the constant coefficient b_0 has a value of 2.0, and the slope coefficient b_1 a value of 0.5.[1] This enables us to write down the straight line equation as:

$$y = 2.0 + 0.5x$$

The value of b_1 of +0.5 is the amount by which y would change if the value of x *increased* by 1. For example, an increase in x from 2 to 3 will cause y to increase from 3 to 3.5, an increase of 0.5.

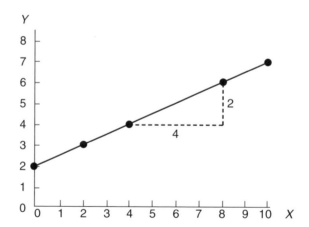

Figure 17.1: A plot of y against and x for the values shown in the text produces a straight line

---

[1] If you draw a right-angled triangle with the straight line forming the hypotenuse, the the slope is equal to the vertical height of the triangle divided by the horizontal distance. The triangle can be of any size (bigger is better) and anywhere along the line; e.g. 2/4 = 0.5.

THE STRAIGHT LINE, THE RELATIONSHIP, AND THE LINEAR REGRESSION MODEL

In Figure 17.1, all of the points lie *exactly* on the straight line. Outside of a laboratory, this won't happen. Figure 17.2 is an example of what you might see in practice. It is a scatterplot using real data of body mass index in kg/m² and hip circumference in cm, for 412 women selected at random from a large cohort study started in 1996 into the relationship between diet and health, and involving over 36,000 British women.[2] Our objective here is to determine whether and how body mass index (BMI) is related to hip circumference, *assuming* that there is a potential relationship with changes in the circumference *causing* changes in BMI. In particular we need to establish that the relationship is linear if we are to use the linear regression model. One way is to examine the scatterplot in Figure 17.2.

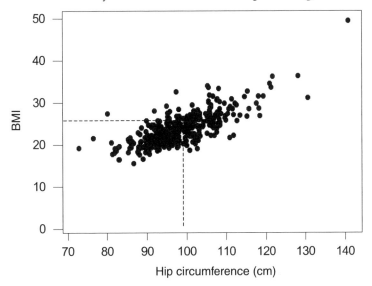

Figure 17.2: Scatterplot of body mass index (kg/m²) against hip circumference (cm), for 412 women in a diet and health cohort study. Each dot represents one woman, and they appear to be distributed around a straight line. That is, the relationship appears to be broadly linear

The points in the scatterplot do *seem* to cluster close to a straight line, sloping upwards from left to right, indicating a possible linear relationship. The equation of the corresponding imaginary line in the population can be used to *model* this relationship.[3] We call this model the *population linear regression model*, and write it as follows:

$$BMI = \beta_0 + \beta_1 \times Hip.$$

The variable on the left-hand side of the equation, *BMI*, is known variously as the outcome, response, or dependent variable[4], and is actually the population *mean*

---

[2] Thanks to Janet Cade for this data.

[3] The word "model" simply means to express a relationship with a mathematical equation. For example, $e = mc^2$ is a model—of the relationship between energy and mass. Claudia Schaeffer is also a model, but of a different sort.

[4] I am going to use the term "dependent variable" in this chapter (and "outcome variable" in the next).

value of BMI for any specified hip measurement. This is an important point and we will return to it in the next chapter. For example, the population *mean* body mass index of all the women with $Hip = 100$cm is about 23kg/m². This dependent variable must be *metric continuous*.

The variable on the right-hand side of the equation, *Hip*, is known variously as the predictor, explanatory, or independent variable, or the covariate. I will use the term "independent variable". This is the variable that's doing the "causing". It is changes in hip circumference that cause body mass index to change in response, but not the other way round. The independent variable can be of any type—nominal, ordinal or metric.

The coefficient β_0 is the population *constant* parameter, and β_1 the population *slope* parameter. I'll return to this example shortly, after a bit of technical stuff. Note that we talk about "regressing *y* on *x*", or "the regression of *y* on *x*", and not the other way round. In theory, *y* can vary from $-\infty$ to $+\infty$, depending on the value of *x*.

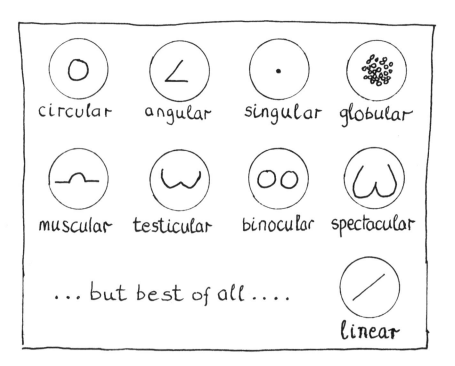

Exercise 17.1

(a) Draw, by eye, the best sample straight line you can through the sample scatterplot in Figure 15.2, and write down the regression equation. What change in mean percentage mortality would you expect if the mean number of episodes per year increased by 1? (b) What is the equation of the regression line shown in Figure 15.5? What value of mean peak viral load would you expect if initial viral load equalled 5? (c) Draw the best straight line you can through the scatterplot in Figure 17.2, and write down the regression equation. By how much would mean body mass index change if mean hip circumference increased by 1cm?

THE METHOD OF ORDINARY LEAST SQUARES (OLS)

You drew the regression line through the scatter of points in Figure 15.2 by eye. Obviously in practice we need a more systematic approach, which will enable us to *calculate* the values of the *sample* coefficients b_0 and b_1.

The most popular method used for this calculation is called *ordinary least squares*, or OLS, and it finds the straight line which best fits the sample data. What do we mean by "best"? It means that if we call the vertical difference between each point in the scatterplot and the straight line the error or *residual* value, e (as shown in Figure 17.3), and if we calculate e^2, the square of each of these residuals, and then add all the e^2 terms together to get the "sum of squares", then the "best" straight line is the one for which this sum is smallest.

BASIC ASSUMPTIONS OF THE LINEAR REGRESSION MODEL

OLS is guaranteed to produce the line of best fit only if the following assumptions are satisfied:

- The relationship between y and x is linear.
- The dependent variable y is metric continuous.
- The residual term, e, is Normally distributed.
- The spread of the residual terms should be the same whatever the value of x. In other words, e shouldn't spread out more (or less) when x increases.

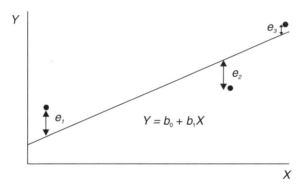

Figure 17.3: The three residual terms for three subjects, used in the method of ordinary least squares. The "best" straight line is the one for which the sum of all the e^2 terms is the smallest

Let me explain the last two assumptions. Suppose you had 50 women with a hip circumference of 100cm. As the scatterplot in Figure 17.2 indicates, most of these women have a different BMI. As you know, the difference between each individual woman's BMI and the regression line are the residuals e. If you arranged these 50 residual values into a frequency distribution, then the third assumption stipulates that this distribution should be Normal.

The fourth assumption demands that if you repeated the above exercise for each separate value of hip circumference, then the spreads (the standard deviations) of each distribution of residual values should be the same, for all hip sizes. If the residual terms have this latter property they are said to be *homoskedastic*.

These assumptions may seem complicated, but the consequences for the accuracy of the ordinary least squares estimators may be serious if they are violated. Needless to say, these assumptions should be checked. I'll return to this later.

BACK TO THE EXAMPLE . . .

The first thing you should do is inspect a scatterplot of your two variables, to check that the relationship is linear, which we did with Figure 17.2. Pearson's correlation coefficient for the two variables is 0.784 (p-value = 0.000), so they are positively and significantly associated. The next thing is to use an appropriate computer program to calculate b_0 and b_1, the OLS estimates of β_0 and β_1, together with their confidence intervals and/or p-values, which will enable you to assess their statistical significance.

The *null hypothesis* is that β_0 and β_1 are each equal to 0 in the population. In practice we have very little interest in the constant coefficient β_0—it's only there to keep a mathematical equality between the left- and right-hand sides of the equation, and in reality it often has no sensible interpretation. For example, in the current example, β_0 would equal the BMI of individuals with a hip circumference equal to 0!

If β_1 is not statistically significant (i.e. it has a confidence interval which includes 0, or a p-value greater than 0.05), then you *cannot* reject the null hypothesis that β_1 is equal to 0. In which case, hip circumference cannot possibly affect body mass index since, whatever its value, once multiplied by 0 it disappears from the regression equation. So the focus in linear regression analysis is *to estimate the value of β_1 and examine its statistical significance*. If β_1 is statistically significant, then the relationship is established (well, at least with a confidence level of 95%).

Using SPSS
If you use the SPSS linear regression program with the data on the 412 women in Figure 17.2, you will get the output shown in Figure 17.4. SPSS provides both a p-value and a 95% confidence interval.

Using Minitab
With Minitab you get the output shown in Figure 17.5. Minitab calculates only the p-value, otherwise the results are the same as for SPSS.

Between them, Figures 17.4 and 17.5 provide us with the estimates b_0 and b_1, their 95% confidence intervals, and their p-values, along with a value for R^2 (see below). These results are summarised in Table 17.1. The 95% confidence interval and the p-value is shown alongside each sample coefficient. Both parameters are statistically significant, since neither confidence interval includes 0, and both p-values are less than 0.05. The value of +0.351 for b_1 means that, for every unit (1cm) increase in hip circumference, sample mean BMI will increase by 0.351kg/m^2.

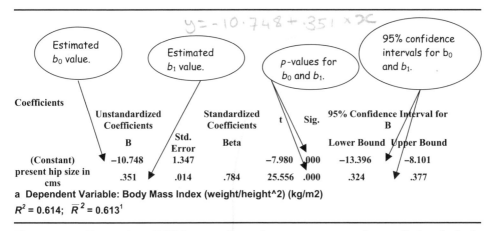

$y = -10.748 + .351 \times x$

Coefficients	Unstandardized Coefficients		Standardized Coefficients	t	Sig.	95% Confidence Interval for B	
	B	Std. Error	Beta			Lower Bound	Upper Bound
(Constant)	−10.748	1.347		−7.980	.000	−13.396	−8.101
present hip size in cms	.351	.014	.784	25.556	.000	.324	.377

a Dependent Variable: Body Mass Index (weight/height^2) (kg/m2)

$R^2 = 0.614$; $\bar{R}^2 = 0.613$[1]

Figure 17.4: Output from SPSS for an ordinary least squares regression applied to the body mass index/hip circumference example. Values for R^2 and $\bar{R}^2$ appear in a separate table in the SPSS output, but for convenience I have copied them to this table

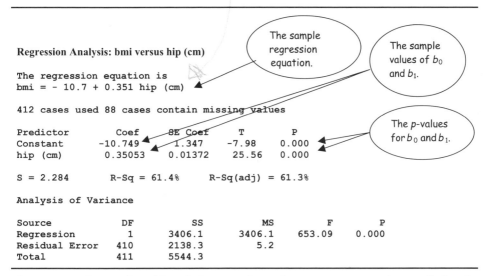

```
Regression Analysis: bmi versus hip (cm)

The regression equation is
bmi = - 10.7 + 0.351 hip (cm)

412 cases used 88 cases contain missing values

Predictor        Coef       SE Coef       T          P
Constant        -10.749     1.347       -7.98      0.000
hip (cm)         0.35053    0.01372     25.56      0.000

S = 2.284        R-Sq = 61.4%      R-Sq(adj) = 61.3%

Analysis of Variance

Source           DF        SS          MS         F         P
Regression       1         3406.1      3406.1     653.09    0.000
Residual Error   410       2138.3      5.2
Total            411       5544.3
```

Figure 17.5: Output from Minitab for an ordinary least squares regression applied to the body mass index/hip circumference example

Table 17.1 Output from the regression of *BMI* on *Hip*

DEPENDENT VARIABLE	COEFFICIENT	ESTIMATED VALUE	95% CI	(p-VALUE)	R^2	$\bar{R}^2$
BMI	b_0	−10.748	(−13.396 to −8.101)	0.000		
	b_1	0.351	(0.324 to 0.377)	0.000	61.4%	61.3%

Knowing the equation, you can if you wish draw the estimated regression line on to the scatterplot.

The regression equation also enables us to *predict* the value of mean BMI for any value of hip circumference *within* the range of the sample hip circumference values (71cm to 140cm). For example, for individuals with a hip circumference of 100cm, you can substitute $Hip = 100$ into the sample regression equation and thus calculate a value for a mean BMI of $24.4kg/m^2$. Prediction of BMI for hip circumference values outside the original sample data range requires a more complex procedure which will not be discussed here.

Exercise 17.2
What does the model predict for mean BMI for women with a hip circumference of 150cm?

GOODNESS OF FIT (R^2)

Suppose you think that waist circumference might also be used in place of BMI as a measure of obesity, so you repeat the above procedure but using waist circumference (Wst) as your independent variable instead of Hip. Your results indicate that b_1 is again statistically significant. Now you have two models, in both of which the independent variable has a statistically significant linear relationship with BMI. But which model is best?

In fact the best model is the one which "explains" the greatest proportion of the observed variation in BMI—that is, has the best *goodness of fit*. To put it another way, it's the model whose regression line is, overall, closest to the points in the scatter diagram. One such measure of this explanatory power is known as the *coefficient of determination*, and is denoted R^2.

As a matter of interest, $R^2 = 0.614$ (61.4%) for the hip circumference model, and 0.501 (50.1%) for the waist circumference model. So variation in hip circumference explains 61% of the observed variation in BMI, while variation in waist circumference explains only 50% of the variation. So using hip circumference as your independent variable gives you a better-fitting model.

Here's a thought. If only 61% of the variation in BMI is explained by variation in hip circumference, what is the remaining 39% explained by? One possibility is that the rest is due to chance, to random effects. A more likely possibility is that, as well as hip circumference, there are other variables which contribute something to the variation in BMI; it would be naïve to believe that variation in BMI, or any clinical variable, can be totally explained by just one variable. Which brings us to the *multiple* linear regression model.

MULTIPLE LINEAR REGRESSION

A simple linear regression model is one with only one independent variable on the right-hand side. When you have *more* than one independent variable the regression model is called a *multiple linear regression model*. For example, having noticed that both hip and waist circumference are each significantly related to BMI, you might include them *both* as independent variables. This gives the following model:

$$BMI = \beta_0 + \beta_1 \times Hip + \beta_2 \times Wst.$$

If you use SPPS to derive the ordinary least squares estimators of this model, you get the output shown in Table 17.2. Both b_1 and b_2 are statistically significant, neither confidence interval includes 0. Goodness of fit has improved marginally, R^2 has increased from 61.4% to 63.7%. Note that in the multiple linear regression model, R^2 measures the explanatory power of *all* of the variables currently in the model, acting together.

Table 17.2 Multiple linear regression output from SPSS for a model with body mass index as the dependent variable and both hip and waist circumferences as independent variables

MODEL (dependent variable)	VARIABLE	ESTIMATED COEFFICIENT	95% CI	(P-VALUE)	R^2	$\bar{R}^2$
1 (*BMI*)	Constant	$b_0 = -10.748$	−13.396 to −8.101	0.000		
	Hip	$b_1 = 0.351$	0.324 to 0.377	0.000	61.4%	61.3%
2 (*BMI*)	Constant	$b_0 = -9.645$	−12.250 to −7.041	0.000		
	Hip	$b_1 = 0.261$	0.219 to 0.303	0.000		
	Waist	$b_2 = 0.105$	0.065 to 0.144	0.000	63.7%	63.5%

Dealing with Nominal Independent Variables: Design Variables and Coding

In linear regression most of the independent variables are likely to be metric, or at least ordinal. However, any independent variable which is *nominal* must be *coded* into a so-called *design* (or *dummy*) variable, before being entered into a model. There is only space for a brief description of the process. As an example, suppose in a study of hypertension, with systolic blood pressure (SBP) as your dependent variable, you have age and smoking status (*Smk*) as your independent variables, with *Smk* (a nominal variable) having the categories non-smoker, ex-smoker, and current smoker. This gives the model:

$$y = \beta_0 + \beta_1 \, Age + \beta_2 \, Smk.$$

To enter *Smk* into your computer you would have to score the three categories in some way—but how? As 1, 2, 3, or as 0, 1, 3, etc.—as you can imagine the scores you attribute to each category will affect your results. The answer is to *code* these *three* categories into *two* design variables. Note that the number of design variables is always one less than the number of categories in the variable being coded. In this example, we set out the coding design as in Table 17.3.

So you replace smoking status (with its dodgy numbering) with two new design variables, D_1 and D_2, which take the values in Table 17.3, according to smoking status. The model now becomes:

$$y = \beta_0 + \beta_1 \, Age + \beta_2 D_1 + \beta_3 D_2.$$

For example, if the subject is a current smoker, $D_1 = 1$ and $D_2 = 0$; if an ex-smoker, $D_1 = 0$ and $D_2 = 1$; if a non-smoker, $D_1 = 0$ and $D_2 = 0$. Notice in the last situation that the smoking status variable effectively disappears from the model.

Table 17.3 Coding design for a nominal variable
with three categories

	DESIGN VARIABLE VALUES	
	D_1	D_2
Smoking status		
Non-smoker	0	0
Ex-smoker	0	1
Current smoker	1	0

This coding scheme can be extended to deal with nominal variables with any reasonable number of categories (4, 5, 6?), depending on the sample size.[5] The simplest situation is a nominal variable with only *two* categories, such as sex, which is represented by one design variable with values 0 (if male), or 1 (if female).

Building the Regression Model

There are a number of ways of building a regression model, but the following is one of the more common approaches.

- Identify a list of independent variables that you think might influence your dependent variable. You should include variables on the basis of previous work (your own or that of other researchers), theoretical considerations, the opinions and clinical experience of knowledgeable colleagues, anecdotal reports, feedback from patients, intuition, gut feeling, and so on. If in doubt, include it! Identify the type of each variable on your list.
- Draw a scatterplot and perform a simple linear regression of your dependent variable against each variable on your list separately (these are called *univariate regressions*). Remember that some of these variables might be design variables. Examine the scatter for linearity, and note the *p*-value or confidence interval for the slope coefficient. If any of the scatterplots show a strong but not a linear relationship with the dependent variable, you will need to code them first before entering them into the data sheet. For example you might find that the relationship between the dependent variable and *Age* is strong but not linear. One approach is to group the *Age* values into four groups, based on its three quartile values, and then code the groups with three design variables.
- From the univariate regressions in the previous step, discard all of those variables with a *p*-value of greater than 0.2 (you want to be generous in your selection criteria). Note that even if only one design variable is statistically significant in the univariate regression, you must include the other design variables from its set. Select from the amended list the independent variable which has the smallest *p*-value. Perform a regression analysis with this variable only. Note its coefficient value. This is your starting model.
- Now add to your starting model the next most statistically significant variable from the list. Examine the statistical significance of the added and the existing

---

[5] As a rule of thumb, you need at the very least 10 subjects for each independent variable in your model. If you've got say five ordinal and/or metric independent variables in your model, you would need a minimum of 50 subjects. If you want also to include a single nominal variable with five categories (i.e. four design variables), you would need another 40 subjects. In these circumstances, it might help to amalgamate some categories.

variable. If the new variable is not statistically significant drop it, *unless* there is a noticeable change in the coefficient of the existing variable, in which case retain it, because such a change indicates that it might be a confounder.
- Repeat this process for each variable in your list, dropping those that are, or become, not statistically significant, unless there are coefficient changes. The end of this process is your final model.[6]

The process described above is known as *forward selection*. An alternative procedure is *backwards elimination* (not as painful as it sounds), in which *all* the eligible variables are included as a first step, and then removed one at a time (largest *p*-value first), noting the new statistical significances of the variables left in the model, and any noticeable coefficient changes, as before. A third method offered by most computer programs is *stepwise regression*. In this approach the computer takes over the variable selection process. One problem with this is the loss of control over the process (messing about subtracting and adding variables to a model and observing the changes often enhances one's understanding of the underlying processes), as well as the omission of possible confounders, which may not by themselves be statistically significant.

Goodness of Fit Again ($\bar{R}^2$)

When you add an extra variable to an existing model and want to compare goodness of fits, you need to compare not R^2 but *adjusted* R^2, denoted $\bar{R}^2$. The reasons need not concern us here, but from Figure 17.4 or Figure 17.5, $\bar{R}^2 = 0.613$ in the *simple* regression model with only hip circumference as an independent variable. From Table 17.2, with both hip and waist circumferences included, $\bar{R}^2$ increases to 0.635, so this multiple regression model does show a real improvement in goodness of fit, and would be preferred to either of the simple regression models. Of course you might decide to explore the possibility that other independent variables might also have a significant role to play in explaining variation in body mass index: age is one obvious contender, and should be included in the model.

Exercise 17.3
Table 17.4 contains the results of a multiple linear regression model from a 1998 cross-section study of disability among 1971 adults aged 65 and over in 1986. The objective of the study was to describe the utilisation rates, by elderly people resident in communal establishments, of general practitioners' time. The dependent variable was the *natural log* of weekly utilisation (minutes) per resident.[7] There were 10 independent variables, as shown in the table. (a) Identify those independent variables whose relationship with the dependent variable is statistically significant. (b) What is the effect on the natural log of utilisation time, and what is this in actual minutes, if there is an increase of (i) one person in the number in a private residential home, (ii) one unit in the severity of disability score? (c) How much of the variation in general practitioners' utilisation time is explained by this model?

---

[6] This is sometimes called the *main-effects model*. You might then want to consider the inclusion of interactive variables. Unfortunately I don't have the space to discuss these.
[7] Probably because the researchers believed the utilisation rate to be skewed. See Figure 5.6 for an example of transformed data.

Table 17.4 Sample regression coefficients from a linear regression model, where the dependent variable is the natural logarithm of the utilisation time (minutes) of GPs by elderly patients in residential care, and the independent variables are as shown

EXPLANATORY VARIABLE	β COEFFICIENT (SE)	p-VALUE
Constant	0.073 (0.353)	0.873
Age	<0.0005 (0.004)	0.923
Male sex	0.024 (0.060)	0.685
Severity of disability	0.043 (0.005)	<0.0001
Mental disorders	0.120 (0.061)	0.047
Nervous system disorders	0.116 (0.062)	0.063
Circulatory system disorders	0.122 (0.066)	0.063
Respiratory system disorders	0.336 (0.115)	0.003
Digestive system disorders	0.057 (0.070)	0.415
Type of accommodation:		
Local authority	—	—
Voluntary residential home	−0.084 (0.183)	0.649
Voluntary nursing home	0.562 (0.320)	0.079
Private residential home	−0.173 (0.157)	0.272
Private nursing home	0.443 (0.228)	0.053
Size of establishment (no. of residents)		
Local authority	−0.004 (0.003)	0.170
Voluntary residential home	−0.004 (0.002)	0.069
Voluntary nursing home	−0.002 (0.002)	0.245
Private residential home	0.006 (0.002)	0.017
Private nursing home	−0.007 (0.007)	0.362

$R^2 = 0.1098$; $F_{(17,415)} = 9.71$; $p \leq 0.0001$; sample size = 1971 in 433 sampling units.

Adjustment and Confounding

One of the most attractive features of the multiple regression model is its ability to *adjust* for the effects of possible association between the independent variables— it's quite possible that two or more of the independent variables in a multiple regression model will be associated. For example, hip (*Hip*) and waist (*Wst*) circumference are significantly positively associated ($r = +0.783$; p-value = 0.000). The consequence of such interactions is that if *Hip* increases, *Wst* is also likely to increase. The increase in *Hip* will cause *BMI* to increase both directly, but also indirectly via *Wst*. In these circumstances it's difficult to tell how much of the increase in BMI index is due *directly* to an increase in *Hip*, and how much to the *indirect* effect of an associated increase in *Wst*.

The beauty of the regression model is that each regression coefficient measures only the *direct* effect of its independent variable on the dependent variable, and *controls* or *adjusts* for any possible interaction from any of the other variables in the model. In terms of the results in Table 17.2, an increase in *Hip* of 1cm will cause mean BMI to increase by 0.261kg/m^2 (the value of b_1), and *all* of this increase is caused by the change in hip circumference (plus the inevitable random error). Any effect that a concomitant change in waist circumference might have is adjusted for. The same applies to the value of 0.105 for b_2.

We can use the adjustment property to deal with confounders in just the same way. You will recall that a confounding variable has to be associated with *both* another independent variable *and* the dependent variable (see the discussion in Chapter 6). Notice that the coefficient b_1, which was 0.351 in the simple regression model with *Hip* the only independent variable, decreases to 0.261 with two independent variables. A marked change like this in the coefficient of a variable already in the model when a new variable is added is an indication that one of the variables is a confounder. As you have already seen in the model-building discussion above, in these circumstances both variables should be retained in the model.

An Example from Practice

Table 17.5 is from a cross-section study into the relationship between bone lead and blood lead levels, and the development of hypertension in 512 individuals selected from a cohort study. The table shows the outcome from three multiple linear regression models with systolic blood pressure as the dependent variable. The first model includes blood lead as an independent variable, along with six possible confounding variables.[8] The second and third models were the same as the first model except tibia and patella lead, respectively, were substituted for blood lead. The results include 95% confidence intervals and the R^2 for each model.

Table 17.5 Multiple regression results from a cross-section study into the relationship between bone lead and blood lead levels and the development of hypertension in 512 individuals selected from a cohort study. The figure shows the outcome from three multiple linear regression models, with systolic blood pressure as the dependent variable

VARIABLE	BASELINE MODEL + BLOOD LEAD		BASELINE MODEL + TIBIA LEAD		BASELINE MODEL + PATELLA LEAD	
	Parameter estimate	95% CI	Parameter estimate	95% CI	Parameter estimate	95% CI
Intercept	128.34		125.90		127.23	
Age (years)	0.46*	0.28, 0.64	0.39*	0.20, 0.58	0.44*	0.26, 0.63
Age squared (years²)	−0.02*	−0.04, −0.00	−0.02*	−0.04, −0.00	−0.02*	−0.04, −0.00
Body mass index (kg/m²)	0.36*	0.01, 0.72	0.33	−0.02, 0.69	0.35	−0.00, 0.71
Family history of hypertension (yes/no)	4.36*	1.42, 7.30	4.36*	1.47, 7.25	4.32*	1.42, 7.22
Alcohol intake (g/day)	0.08*	0.00, 0.149	0.07	−0.00, 0.14	0.07	−0.00, 0.14
Calcium intake (10 mg/day)	−0.04*	−0.08, −0.00	−0.04*	−0.07, −0.00	−0.04	−0.07, −0.00
Blood lead (SD)†	−0.13	−1.35, 1.09				
Tibia lead (SD)†			1.37*	0.02, 2.73		
Patella lead (SD)†					0.57	−0.71, 1.84
Model R^2	0.0956		0.1015		0.0950	

* $p < 0.05$.
† Parameter estimates are based on 1 standard deviation (SD) in blood lead level (4.03 µg/dl), tibia lead level (13.65 µg/g), and patella lead level (19.55 µg/g).

As the table shows, the tibia lead model has the best goodness of fit ($R^2 = 0.1015$), but even this model explains only 10% of the observed variation in systolic blood

---

[8] The inclusion of *Age²* in the model is probably an attempt to establish the linearity of the relationship between systolic blood pressure and age. If the coefficient for *Age²* is not statistically significant, then the relationship is probably linear.

pressure. However, this is the only model which supports the relationship between hypertension and lead levels; the 95% confidence interval for tibia lead (0.02 to 2.73) does not include 0. The only confounders statistically significant in all three models are age, family history of hypertension, and calcium intake.

Exercise 17.4
From Table 17.5, which independent variables are statistically significant in all three models? (b) Explain the 95% confidence interval of (0.28 to 0.64) for age in the blood lead model. (c) In which model does a unit (1 year) increase in age change systolic blood pressure the most?

DIAGNOSTICS: CHECKING THE BASIC ASSUMPTIONS

You saw above that ordinary least squares will produce the best estimators only if the basic assumptions of the model are satisfied, that is: a linear relationship, a metric continuous dependent variable, error terms Normally distributed, and with constant spread. All four assumptions can be checked graphically in both SPSS and Minitab, with plots of the residual terms against the fitted values of *BMI* (these latter are the values the estimated regression equation would give for mean *BMI* for every value of *Hip* and *Wst* in their respective sample ranges). Possible outcomes from such a plot are shown in Figure 17.6.

If the relationship between the variables is linear (as required by the first assumption), the scatter of points should be randomly and evenly spread around the zero line as in Figure 17.6(a). If the relationship is non-linear, the scatter of points would be curved in some way. If the spread of the residual terms is constant (as required by the fourth assumption), the spread of the values in the scatter of points shouldn't get wider (or narrower) as the fitted value increases. Non-constant variance might look like Figure 17.6(b). A combination of non-linearity and non-constant variance might produce a scatter of points like Figure 17.6(c). The Normality of the residuals (as required by the third assumption) can be checked by plotting a histogram of the values.

An Example from Practice

For the body mass index model with both hip and waist circumferences included, Minitab produces the plot of the residuals against the fitted *BMI* values shown in Figure 17.7. The distribution of points above and below the 0 line seems reasonably symmetric, implying that the relationships in the model are linear (first assumption). The spread of points across the range of values for fitted BMI seems reasonably uniform, indicating constant spread of the residuals (fourth assumption)

You can check the Normality of the residuals (third assumption) by plotting a histogram of their values. The histogram in Figure 17.8 indicates that, apart from a rather worrying outlier, the distribution is Normal. You might want to identify which woman this outlier represents and check her data for anomalies. Thus all of the basic assumptions appear to be reasonably well satisfied, and the OLS regression parameter estimates b_0 and b_1

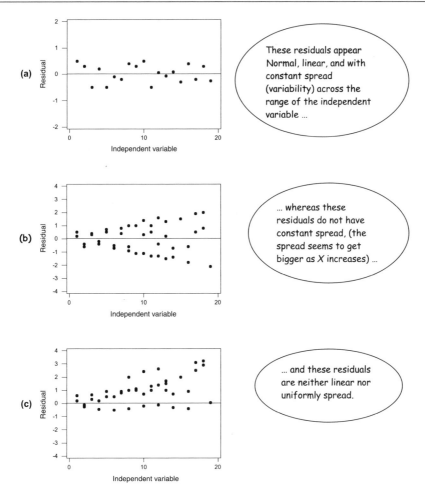

Figure 17.6: Testing the basic assumptions of the linear regression model by plotting the residuals against the fitted values of the regression equation

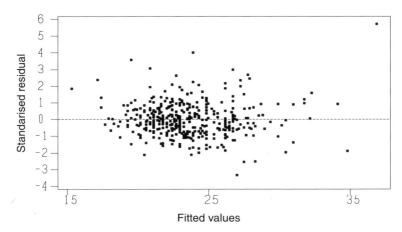

Figure 17.7: Plot of the residuals versus the fitted BMI values as a check of the basic assumptions of the linear regression model

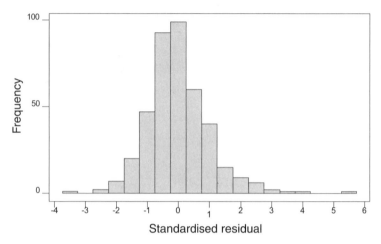

Figure 17.8:   Plot of the residuals in the body mass index example, showing approximate Normality

you obtained fit the data at least as well as any other estimates.[9] Multiple linear regression is moderately popular in clinical research. Much more popular is logistic regression for reasons which will be clearer in the next chapter.

ANALYSIS OF VARIANCE

Analysis of variance (ANOVA) is a procedure which aims to deal with the same problems as linear regression analysis, and many medical statistics books contain at least one chapter describing ANOVA. However, regression and ANOVA are simply two sides of the same coin—the *generalised linear model*. In view of the fact that anything ANOVA can do, regression can also do—and, for me anyway, do it in a way that's conceptually easier—I am not going to discuss ANOVA in this book.

---

[9] There are other methods of estimating the values of the regression parameters, which I don't have the space to consider. However, provided the basic assumptions are satisfied, none will be better than the ordinary least squares estimators.

18

CURVY MODELS: LOGISTIC REGRESSION

Learning objectives

When you have finished this chapter you should be able to:

- *Explain why a linear regression model is not appropriate if the dependent variable is binary*
- *Explain what the logit transformation is and what it achieves*
- *Write down the logic regression equation*
- *Explain the concept of linearity, and outline how this can be tested for and dealt with*
- *Explain how estimates of the odds ratios can be derived directly from the regression parameters*
- *Describe how the statistical significance of the population odds ratio is determined*
- *Interpret output from SPSS and Minitab logistic regression programs*

A Second Health Warning!

Although the maths underlying the logistic regression model is perhaps more complicated than in linear regression, a brief description of the underlying idea is necessary if you are to gain any understanding at all of the procedure and be able to interpret logistic computer outputs sensibly. I have tried to keep the maths as simple as possible, but despite this some stuff is unavoidable. You may want to skip straight to equation (8).

BINARY DEPENDENT VARIABLES

In linear regression the dependent or outcome variable must be metric continuous. In clinical research, however, the outcome variable in a relationship will very often be dichotomous or *binary*. That means it can take only *two* different values—alive or dead, malignant or benign, admitted or discharged, and so on. In addition, variables which are not naturally binary can often be made so. For example, birthweight might be coded "less than 2500g" and "2500g or more", Apgar scores coded "less than 7" and "7 or more", etc. In this chapter I want to show how a binary dependent variable makes the linear regression model inappropriate, and suggest an alternative approach.

FINDING AN APPROPRIATE MODEL WHEN THE OUTCOME VARIABLE IS BINARY

If you are trying to find an appropriate model to describe the relationship between two variables y and x, when y, the dependent or outcome variable, is continuous, you can draw a scatterplot of y against x (Figure 17.2 is a good example), and if this has a linear shape you can model the relationship with the linear regression model. However, when the outcome variable is binary, this graphical approach may not be particularly helpful.

For example, suppose you are interested in using the breast cancer/stress data to investigate the relationship between the outcome variable "Diagnosis" and the independent variable "Age". Diagnosis is of course a binary variable with two values: $y = 1$ (malignant) or $y = 0$ (benign). If we plot diagnosis against age, we get the scatterplot shown in Figure 18.1, from which it's difficult to draw any definite conclusions about the nature of the relationship!

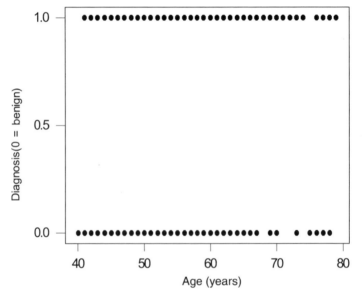

Figure 18.1:   Scatterplot of diagnosis against age for the 332 women in the breast cancer–stress study referred to in Table 1.2

The problem is that the large variability in age in both the malignant and benign groups obscures the difference (if any) between them. However, if you *group* the age data into groups 40–49, 50–59, etc., and then calculate the *proportion* of women with a malignant diagnosis (i.e. with $y = 1$), in each group, this will reduce the variability but preserve the underlying relationship between the two variables. The results of doing this are shown in Table 18.1.

Notice that the first column stipulates the proportion with $y = 1$, *or* the probability that $y = 1$, written as $p(y = 1)$. Here's why. In linear regression you will recall that the dependent variable is the *mean* of y for a given x. But the mean of a binary, 0 or 1, variable is the same as the *proportion* of 1s (see p. 42). So an appropriate dependent variable would seem to be the proportion of $y = 1$s. But proportions

Table 18.1:   Proportion of women with a malignant lump, in each age group

PROPORTION WITH MALIGNANT LUMP*	MIDPOINT OF AGE GROUP
0.140	45
0.226	55
0.635	65
0.727	75

*That is, $y = 1$ or $p(y = 1)$. See the text for an explanation.

can be interpreted as probabilities (see Table 8.1), so the dependent variable becomes the probability that $y = 1$, or $p(y = 1)$, for a given value of x.[1]

You can see in Table 18.1 that the proportion with malignant breast lumps (the probability that $y = 1$) increases with age, but does it increase linearly? A scatterplot of the proportion with malignant lumps, $y = 1$, against group age midpoints is shown in Figure 18.2, which does suggest *some* sort of relationship between the two variables, but it's definitely *not* linear, so a *linear* regression model won't work. In fact, the curve has more of an S-shape, rather like a cumulative frequency curve or ogive, so what you need is a mathematical format which will give an S-shaped curve. There are several possibilities, but the *logistic regression model* is the model of choice, not only because it produces an S-shaped curve, but, critically, it has a meaningful clinical interpretation. Moreover, the value of $p(y = 1)$ is restricted by the maths of the logistic model to lie between 0 and 1, which is what we want since it's a probability.

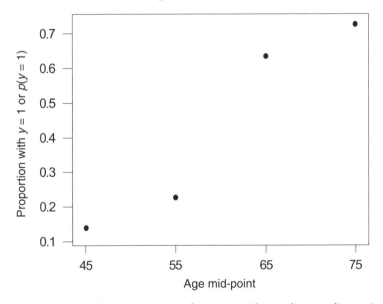

Figure 18.2:   Scatterplot of the proportion of women with a malignant diagnosis, $y = 1$, in each age group against midpoints of the age group

---

[1] For example, the probability of a malignant diagnosis ($y = 1$) for a woman who is, say, aged 40; i.e. $x = 40$.

The *simple* logistic regression model has the following form:

$$P(y = 1) = (e^{b_0 + b_1 x})/(1 + e^{b_0 + b_1 x}). \tag{1}$$

The outcome variable, $P(y = 1)$, is the probability that $y = 1$ (e.g. the lump is malignant), for some given value of the independent variable x. There is no restriction on the type of *independent* variable, which can be nominal, ordinal or metric. In a simple logistic model such as this we might use a suspected risk factor as our independent variable. For example, if lung cancer (Y or N) is the outcome variable, then the independent variable might be the *risk factor* smoking (Y or N).

Let's stick with our breast cancer example, with the outcome variable "Diagnosis", $y = 1$ (malignant) $y = 0$ (benign); and with the independent variable "Ever used an oral contraceptive pill" (*OCP*), yes = 1, or no = 0. We are going to treat OCP use as a possible risk factor for receiving a malignant diagnosis. So all we've got to do to determine the probability that a woman picked at random from the sample will get a malignant diagnosis ($y = 1$) is to calculate the values of b_0 and b_1, somehow, and then put them in the logistic regression equation, with the appropriate value of x, i.e. either 0 or 1. Note, however, that if $x = 1$ (woman has used an OCP), equation (1) becomes:

$$P(y = 1) = (e^{b_0 + b_1})/(1 + e^{b_0 + b_1}). \tag{2}$$

If $x = 0$ (woman has never used an OCP), equation (1) becomes:

$$P(y = 1) = (e^{b_0})/(1 + e^{b_0}). \tag{3}$$

We will use these results again when we see how we can readily get an odds ratio out of a logistic regression.

Estimating the Parameter Values

Whereas the linear regression models use the method of ordinary least squares to estimate the regression parameters b_0 and b_1, logistic regression models use what is called *maximum-likelihood estimation*. Essentially this means choosing the population which is most likely to have generated the sample results observed. As an example, let's use data from the breast cancer/stress study again and the relationship between the outcome variable "Diagnosis" and the binary independent variable, "Ever used an oral contraceptive pill".

Figures 18.3 and 18.4 respectively, show the outputs from SPSS's and Minitab's logistic regression programs for the OCP model. Both programs give $b_0 = -0.2877$ and $b_1 = -0.9507$. If we substitute these values into the logistic regression model of equation (1), or directly into equations (2) and (3), we get:

> If $x = 1$ (has used an OCP), $p(y = 1) = 0.2247$
> If $x = 0$ (has never used an OCP), $p(y = 1) = 0.4286$.

So a woman who has never used an oral contraceptive pill has a probability of getting a malignant diagnosis nearly twice that of a woman who *has* used an oral

Logistic Regression

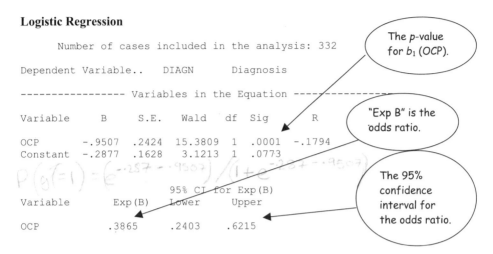

```
        Number of cases included in the analysis: 332

Dependent Variable..    DIAGN        Diagnosis

----------------- Variables in the Equation ----------------

Variable      B       S.E.    Wald    df   Sig            R

OCP        -.9507    .2424  15.3809    1  .0001       -.1794
Constant   -.2877    .1628   3.1213    1  .0773


                           95% CI for Exp(B)
Variable       Exp(B)    Lower      Upper

OCP            .3865     .2403      .6215
```

The p-value for b₁ (OCP).

"Exp B" is the odds ratio.

The 95% confidence interval for the odds ratio.

Figure 18.3: Abbreviated output from SPSS for a logistic regression with diagnosis as the dependent variable and use of oral contraceptive pill (OCP) as the independent variable or risk factor

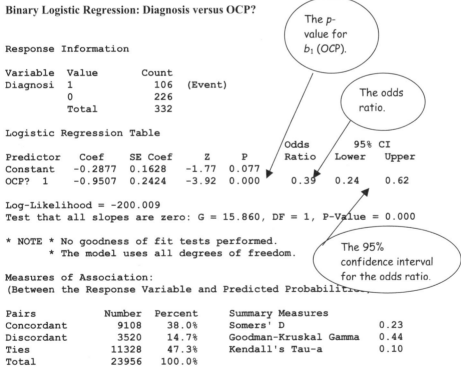

Binary Logistic Regression: Diagnosis versus OCP?

The p-value for b₁ (OCP).

The odds ratio.

```
Response Information

Variable  Value        Count
Diagnosi  1              106    (Event)
          0              226
          Total          332

Logistic Regression Table
                                                 Odds         95% CI
Predictor    Coef    SE Coef      Z      P       Ratio    Lower    Upper
Constant   -0.2877   0.1628   -1.77   0.077
OCP?  1    -0.9507   0.2424   -3.92   0.000      0.39     0.24     0.62


Log-Likelihood = -200.009
Test that all slopes are zero: G = 15.860, DF = 1, P-Value = 0.000

* NOTE * No goodness of fit tests performed.
       * The model uses all degrees of freedom.

Measures of Association:
(Between the Response Variable and Predicted Probabilitie.

Pairs            Number   Percent    Summary Measures
Concordant         9108    38.0%     Somers' D                  0.23
Discordant         3520    14.7%     Goodman-Kruskal Gamma      0.44
Ties              11328    47.3%     Kendall's Tau-a            0.10
Total             23956   100.0%
```

The 95% confidence interval for the odds ratio.

Figure 18.4: Output from Minitab for a logistic regression with diagnosis as the dependent variable and use of oral contraceptive pill (OCP) as the independent variable or risk factor

contraceptive. Rather than being a risk factor for a malignant diagnosis, in this example use of oral contraceptives seems to confer some protection against malignancy.

Towards the Odds Ratio

The great attraction of the logistic regression model is that it readily produces odds ratios. But to see how we need to do a bit more maths. Recall from Chapter 8 that if p is the probability of an event happening, then $(1 - p)$ is the probability of it not happening. So if $p(y = 1)$ is the probability that $y = 1$, then $[1 - p(y = 1)]$ is the probability that y is *not* equal to 1; i.e. that $p(y = 0)$. If we divide the former probability by the latter, we get:

$$\left\{ \frac{p(y = 1)}{[1 - p(y = 1)]} \right\}.$$

This transformation of $p(y = 1)$ is known as the *logit transformation*, or just the *logit*. But look at the term inside the curly brackets. This has the form: the probability of an event (i.e. the event $y = 1$), divided by 1 minus the probability of the event. Now recall from Chapter 8 that [probability/(1 − probability)] is the *odds* for the event. In this case it is the odds that $y = 1$ (malignant diagnosis) for a given value of x. For example, if $x = 1$, it is the odds that a woman will have a malignant diagnosis if she has used an oral contraceptive; if $x = 0$, it is the odds that she will have a malignant diagnosis if she has not used an OCP. In other words, the term inside the curly brackets is the odds that y will equal 1 (for some given x).

Now we already know the value of $p(y = 1)$ when $x = 1$ and when $x = 0$ from equations (2) and (3). So to calculate the odds we need to determine the value of $[1 - p(y = 1)]$ when $x = 1$ and when $x = 0$; then we can divide $p(y = 1)$ by $[1 - p(y = 1)]$ for each x. This will give us the two sets of odds for $y = 1$, one when $x = 1$ and one when $x = 0$. If we divide these two odds we get the odds ratio.

First from equation (2) we can show that when $x = 1$:

$$[1 - p(y = 1)] = 1/(1 + e^{b_0 + b_1}) \tag{4}$$

and from equation (3) we can show that when $x = 0$:

$$[1 - p(y = 1)] = 1/(1 + e^{b_0}). \tag{5}$$

So the odds for $y = 1$ when $x = 1$ are equal to equation (2) divided by equation (4), which after some algebra becomes:

$$\text{Odds that } y = 1 \text{ when } x = 1 \text{ are } e^{b_0 + b_1} \tag{6}$$

and the odds for $y = 1$ when $x = 0$ are equal to equation (3) divided by equation (5), which after some algebra becomes:

$$\text{Odds that } y = 1 \text{ when } x = 0 \text{ are } e^{b_0}. \tag{7}$$

Thus the odds ratio that $y = 1$ (malignant) when $x = 1$ (used an OCP), compared to when $x = 0$ (no OCP use), is equation (6) divided by (7):

$$\text{Odds ratio} = e^{b_0 + b_1}/e^{b_0} = e^{b_1} \tag{8}$$

It is this ability to produce odds ratios that has made the logistic regression model so popular in clinical studies. Thus to find the odds ratio all you need to do is raise e to the power b_1, easily done on a decent calculator. Now, in our diagnosis/OCP model, $b_0 = -0.2877$ and $b_1 = -0.9507$, so the odds ratio for a malignant diagnosis for woman using an OCP compared to women not using an OCP is:

Odds ratio = $e^{-0.9507}$ = 0.386.

In other words, a woman who has used an OCP has only about a third of the odds of getting a malignant diagnosis as a woman who has not used an OCP. It seems that use of an OCP provides some protection against a malignancy. Of course we don't know whether this result is due to chance, or whether this represents a real statistically significant result in the population. To answer that question we will need either a confidence interval for b_1 or a p-value, which I'll come to shortly.

Interpreting the Regression Coefficient

In linear regression the coefficient b_1 represents the change in y for a unit increase in x. But what does b_1 mean in the logistic regression model? I can answer this question using equation (8) and logarithms. If we take the $\log_e$ of equation (8) we get:

$\log_e$(odds ratio) = $\log_e(e^{b_1})$ = b_1.

This expression is known as the *log odds ratio*, or just the *log-odds*. In other words, a unit increase in x increases the log-odds by the amount b_1 (which may of course be negative or positive). When x is a binary variable, as OCP use is, then b_1 represents the change in the log-odds between a woman who hasn't used an OCP ($x = 0$) and one who has ($x = 1$).

Note that if the independent variable is ordinal or metric, then you might be more interested in the effect on the odds ratio of changes of *greater* than one unit. For example, if the independent variable is age, then the effect on the odds ratio of an increase in age of 1 year may not be as useful as, say, a change of 10 years. In these circumstances, if the change in the independent variable, say age, is c years, then the change in the log$_e$ odds is cb_1, and the change in the odds ratio is therefore e^{cb_1}.

Exercise 18.1
(a) In linear regression we can plot y against x to determine whether the relationship between the two variables is linear. Explain why this approach is not particularly helpful when y is a binary variable. What approach might be more useful? (b) Figure 18.5 shows the output from Minitab for the regression of diagnosis on age for the breast cancer example. Is age a statistically significant risk? Explain. (c) Use the Minitab values to write down the estimated logistic regression model. (d) Calculate the probability that the diagnosis will be malignant, $p(y = 1)$, for women aged (i) 45, and (ii) aged 50. (e) Calculate $[1 - p(y = 1)]$ in each case, and hence calculate the odds ratio for a malignant diagnosis in women aged 45 compared to women aged 50. Explain your result. (f) Confirm that the antilog$_e$ of the coefficient on age is equal to the odds ratio (g) What effect does an increase in age of 10 years have on the odds ratio?

```
Logistic Regression Table. Dependent variable is Diagnosis.
                                                Odds        95% CI
Predictor      Coef    SE Coef      Z      P    Ratio    Lower   Upper
Constant    -6.4672     0.7632   -8.47  0.000
Age          0.10231    0.01326    7.72  0.000   1.11     1.08    1.14
```

Figure 18.5:   Output from Minitab for the logistic regression of diagnosis on age

Statistical Inference in the Logistic Regression Model

As you saw in Chapter 11, if the population odds ratio is equal to 1, the risk factor concerned has no effect on the odds for any particular outcome; that is, the variable concerned is *not* a statistically significant risk (or benefit). In fact the 95% confidence interval for the odds ratio for OCP use and a malignant diagnosis is (0.24 to 0.62), and since this does not include 1, the odds ratio is statistically significant. However, we still need to be cautious about this result because it represents only a crude odds ratio, which in reality would need to be adjusted for other variables, such as age. We can make this adjustment in logistic regression just as easily as in a linear regression model, simply by including the variables we want to adjust for on the right-hand side of the model.

The Multiple Logistic Regression Model

In my explanation of the odds ratio above I used a simple logistic regression model—i.e. one with a single independent variable (*OCP*)—because this offers the

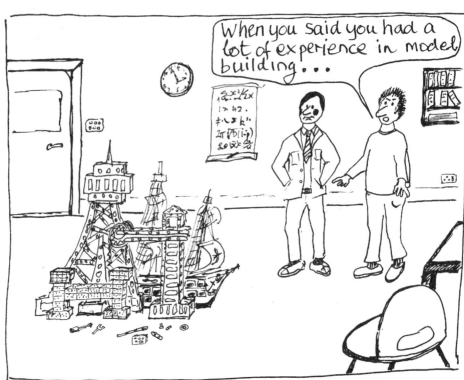

simplest treatment. However the result we got, that the odds ratio is e^{b_1}, applies equally to *each* coefficient if there is more than one independent variable. The usual situation is to have a risk factor variable plus a number of confounder variables (the usual suspects—age, sex, etc.). Suppose, for example, that you decided to include *Age* and body mass index (*BMI*) along with *OCP* as independent variables. Equation (1) would then become:

$$p(y = 1) = (e^{b_0 + b_1 \times OCP + b_2 XAge + b_3 \times BMI})/(1 + e^{b_0 + b_1 \times OCP + b_2 XAge + b_3 \times BMI}).$$

$p(y = 1)$ is still of course the probability that the woman will receive a malignant diagnosis, $y = 1$. The odds ratio for *Age* is e^{b_2}, the odds ratio for *BMI* is e^{b_3}. Moreover, as with linear regression, each of these odds ratios is *adjusted* for any possible interaction between the independent variables. So, whichever variable we want to adjust for we simply include as an independent variable in the model.

BUILDING THE MODEL

The strategy for model building in the logistic regression model is much the same as in linear regression. First make a list of candidate independent variables. Second, for any nominal or ordinal variables in the list construct a contingency-type table and do a chi-squared test.[2] Make a note of the *p*-value. Third, for any metric variables, do either a two-sample *t*-test, or a simple logistic regression, and note the *p*-value in either case. Fourth, pick out all those variables in the list with a *p*-value of 0.25 or less. Select that variable with the smallest *p*-value (if there is more than one with the smallest *p*-value pick one arbitrarily) to be your first independent variable. This is your starting model. Finally, add variables to your model one at a time, each time examining the *p*-values for statistical significance. If a variable when added to the model is not statistically significant, drop it, unless there are noticeable changes in coefficient values, which are indicative of confounding.

GOODNESS OF FIT

In the linear regression model you used R^2 to measure goodness of fit. In the logistic regression model measuring goodness of fit is much more complicated, and can involve graphical as well as numeric measures. Two numeric measures available are the *deviance coefficient* and the *Hosmer–Lemshow statistic*. Very briefly, both of these have a chi-squared distribution, and we can use the resultant *p*-value to reject or not the null hypothesis that the model provides a good fit. The graphical methods are quite complex and you should consult more specialist sources for further information on this and other aspects of this complex procedure. Hosmer and Lemeshow (1989) is an excellent resource.

---

[2] Provided the number of categories isn't too big for the size of your sample—you don't want any empty cells or low expected values (see Chapter 14).

AND FINALLY

Linear and logistic regression modelling are two methods from a class of methods known collectively as *multivariable* statistics. *Multivariate* statistics is applicable where there is more than one dependent variable and comprises a collection of procedures, such as principal component analysis, multidimensional scaling, cluster, and discriminant analysis, and more. Of these, principal components appears most often in the clinical literature, but even so is not very common. Unfortunately, there is no space to discuss any of these methods.

APPENDIX: TABLE OF
RANDOM NUMBERS

23157	54859	01837	25993	76249	70886	95230	36744
05545	55043	10537	43508	90611	83744	10962	21343
14871	60350	32404	36223	50051	00322	11543	80834
38976	74951	94051	75853	78805	90194	32428	71695
97312	61718	99755	30870	94251	25841	54882	10513
11742	69381	44339	30872	32797	33118	22647	06850
43361	28859	11016	45623	93009	00499	43640	74036
93806	20478	38268	04491	55751	18932	58475	52571
49540	13181	08429	84187	69538	29661	77738	09527
36768	72633	37948	21569	41959	68670	45274	83880
07092	52392	24627	12067	06558	45344	67338	45320
43310	01081	44863	80307	52555	16148	89742	94647
61570	06360	06173	63775	63148	95123	35017	46993
31352	83799	10779	18941	31579	76448	62584	86919
57048	86526	27795	93692	90529	56546	35065	32254
09243	44200	68721	07137	30729	75756	09298	27650
97957	35018	40894	88329	52230	82521	22532	61587
93732	59570	43781	98885	56671	66826	95996	44569
72621	11225	00922	68264	35666	59434	71687	58167
61020	74418	45371	20794	95917	37866	99536	19378
97839	85474	33055	91718	45473	54144	22034	23000
89160	97192	22232	90637	35055	45489	88438	16361
25966	88220	62871	79265	02823	52862	84919	54883
81443	31719	05049	54806	74690	07567	65017	16543
11322	54931	42362	34386	08624	97687	46245	23245

BIBLIOGRAPHY

I have referred to the following papers and books in writing this book:

Altgassen C, Possover M, Krause N, Plaul K, Michels W, Schneider A. Establishing a new technique of laporoscopic pelvic and para-aortic lymphadectomy. *Obstet Gynecol* 2000, 95:348–52.

Altman DG. *Practical Statistics for Medical Research*. London: Chapman & Hall, 1991.

Assessment of the Safety and Efficacy of a New Thrombolytic (ASSENT-2) Investigators. *Lancet* 1999, 354:716–21.

Bland JM, Altman DG. Statistical methods for assessing agreement between two clinical measurements. *Lancet* 1986, I:307–10.

Bland M. *An Introduction to Medical Statistics*. Oxford: Oxford University Press, 1995.

Brueren MM, Schouten HJA, de Leeuw PW, van Montfrans GA, van Ree JW. A series of self-measurements by the patient is a reliable alternative to ambulatory blood pressure measurement. *Br J Gen Pract* 1998, 48:1585–9.

Chapman KR, Kesten S, Szalai JP. Regular vs as-needed inhaled salbutamol in asthma control. *Lancet* 1994, 343:1379–83.

Cheng Y, Schartz J, Sparrow D, Aro A, Weiss ST, Hu H. Bone lead and blood lead levels in relation to baseline blood pressure and the prospective development of hypertension. *Am J Epidemiol* 2001, 153:164–71.

Chi-Ling C, Gilbert TJ, Daling JR. Maternal smoking and Down syndrome: the confounding effect of maternal age. *Am J Epidemiol* 1999, 149:442–6.

Chosidow O, Chastang C *et al*. Controlled study of malathion and *d*-phenothrin lotions for *Pediculus humanus* var. *capitas*-infested schoolchildren. *Lancet* 1994, 344:1724–6.

Conter V, Cortinovis I, Rogari P, Riva L. Weight growth in infants born to mothers who smoked during pregnancy. *Br Med J* 1995, 310:768–71.

Cook DG, Whincup PH, Jarvis MJ, Strachan DP, Papacosta O, Bryant A. Passive exposure to tobacco smoke in children aged 5–7 years: individual, family, and community factors. *Br Med J* 1994, 308:384–9.

DeStafano F, Anda RF, Kahn HS, Williamson DF, Russell CM. Dental disease and risk of coronary heart disease and mortality. *Br Med J* 1993, 306:688–91.

Emery VC, Sabin CA, Cope AV, Gor D, Hassan-Walker AF, Griffiths PD. Application of viral load kinetics to identify patients who develop cytomegalovirus disease after transplantation. *Lancet* 2000, 355:3032–6.

Fall CHD, Vijayakumar M, Barker DJP, Osmond C, Duggleby S. Weight in infancy and prevalence of coronary heart disease in adult life. *Br Med J* 1995, 310:17–19.

Fragmin and Fast Revascularisation during Instability in Coronary Artery Disease Investigators. Long-term low-molecular-mass heparin in unstable coronary-artery disease: FRISC II prospective randomised multicentre study. *Lancet* 1999, 354:701–7.

Goel V, Iron K, Williams JI. Enthusiasm or uncertainty: small area variations in the use of the mammography services in Ontario, Canada. *J Epidemiol Comm Health* 1997, 51:378–82.

Grampian Asthma Study of Integrated Care. Integrated care for asthma: a clinical, social, and economic evaluation. *Br Med J* 1994, 308:559–64.

Gronbaek M, Deis A, Sorensen TIA *et al*. Influence of sex, age, body mass index, and smoking on alcohol intake and mortality. *Br Med J* 1994, 308:302–6.

Ham C. Priority setting in the NHS: reports from six districts. *Br Med J* 1993, 307: 435–9.

He Y, Lam TH, Li LS *et al*. Passive smoking at work as a risk factor for coronary heart disease in Chinese women who have never smoked. *Br Med J* 1994, 308:380–84.

Hearn J, Higinson IJ, on behalf of the Palliative Care Core Audit Project Advisory Group. Development and validation of a core outcome measure for palliative care: the palliative care outcome scale. *Qual Health Care* 1998, 8:219–27.

Hosmer DW, Lemeshow S. *Applied Logistic Regression Analysis*. Chichester: Wiley, 1989.

Hu FB, Wand B, Chen C *et al*. Body mass index and cardiovascular risk factors in a rural Chinese population. *Am J Epidemiol* 2000, 151:88–97.

Imperial Cancer Fund. Effectiveness of health checks conducted by nurses in primary care: final results of the OXCHECK study. *Br Med J* 1995, 310:1099–104.

Inzitari D, Eliasziw M, Gates P *et al*. The causes and risk of stroke in patients with asymptotic internal-carotid-artery stenosis. *New Engl J Med* 2000: 342:1693–9.

Kavanagh S, Knapp M. The impact on general practitioners of the changing balance of care for elderly people living in an institution. *Br Med J* 1998, 317:322–7.

Kjerulff KH, Langenberg PW, Rhodes JC, Harvey LA, Guzinski GM, Stolley PD. Effectiveness of hysterectomy. *Obstet Gynecol* 2000, 95:319–26.

Knaus WA, Draper EA, Wagner DP, Zimmerman JE. APACHE II: a severity of disease classification system. *Crit Care Med* 1985, 13:818–29.

Ladwig KH, Roll G, Breithardt G, Budde T, Borggrefe M. Post-infarction depression and incomplete recovery 6 months after acute myocardial infarction. *Lancet* 1994. 343:20–23.

Leeson CPM, Kattenhorn JE, Lucas A. Duration of breast feeding and arterial disability in early adult life: a population based study. *Br Med J* 2001, 322:643–7.

Lindberg G, Bingefors K, Ranstam J, Rastam AM. Use of calcium channel blockers and risk of suicide: ecological findings confirmed in population based cohort study. *Br Med J* 1998, 316:741–5.

Lindelow M, Hardy R, Rodgers B. Development of a scale to measure symptoms of anxiety and depression in the general UK population: the psychiatric symptom frequency scale. *J Epidemiol Comm Health* 1997, 51:549–57.

Lindqvist P, Dahlback MD, Marsal K. Thrombotic risk during pregnancy: a population study. *Obstet Gynecol* 1999, 94:595–9.

Luke A, Durazo-Arvizu R, Rotimi C *et al*. Relations between body mass index and body fat in black population samples from Nigeria, Jamaica, and the United States. *Am J Epidemiol* 1997, 145:620–28.

McCreadie R, Macdonald E, Blacklock C *et al*. Dietary intake of schizophrenic patients in Nithsdale, Scotland: case–control study. *Br Med J* 1998, 317:784–5.

McKee M, Hunter D. Mortality league tables: do they inform or mislead? *Qual Health Care* 1995, 4:5–12.

Machin D, Campbell MJ, Fayers PM, Pinol APY. *Sample Size Tables for Clinical Studies*. Oxford: Blackwell Scientific, 1987.

Michelson D, Stratakis C, Hill L *et al*. Bone mineral density in women with depression. *New Engl J Med* 1996, 335:1176–81.

Nikolajsen L, Ilkjaer S, Christensen JH, Kroner K, Jensen TS. Randomised trial of epidural bupivacaine and morphine in prevention of stump and phantom pain in lower-limb amputation. *Lancet* 1997, 350:1353–7.

Nordentoft M, Breum L, Munck LK, Nordestgaard AH, Bjaeldager PAL. High mortality by natural and unnatural causes: a 10-year follow-up study of patients admitted to a poisoning treatment centre after suicide attempts. *Br Med J* 1993, 306:1637–41.

Olson JE, Shu XO, Ross JA, Pendergrass T, Robison LL. Medical record validation of maternity reported birth characteristics and pregnancy-related events: a report from the Children's Cancer Group. *Am J Epidemiol* 1997, 145:58–67.

Prevots DR, Watson JC, Redd SC, Atkinson WA. Outbreak in highly vaccinated populations: implications for studies of vaccine performance. *Am J Epidemiol* 1997, 146:881–2.

Protheroe D, Turvey K, Horgan K, Benson E, Bowers D, House A. Stressful life events and difficulties and onset of breast cancer: case–control study. *Br Med J* 1999, 319:1027–30.

Rainer TH, Jacobs P, Ng YC *et al*. Cost effectiveness analysis of intravenous ketorolac and morphine for treating pain after limb injury: double blind randomised controlled trail. *Br Med J* 2000, 321:1247–51.

Ramirez AJ, Craig TKJ, Watson JP, Fentiman IS, North WRS, Rubens RD. Stress and relapse of breast cancer. *Br Med J* 1989, 298:291–3.

Relling MV, Rubnitz JE, Rivera GK *et al*. High incidence of secondary brain tumours after radiotherapy and antimetabolites. *Lancet* 1999, 354:34–9.

Rodgers M, Miller JE. Adequacy of hormone replacement therapy for osteoporosis prevention assessed by serum oestradiol measurement, and the degree of association with menopausal symptoms. *Br J Gen Pract* 1997, 47:161–5.

Rogers A, Pilgrim D. Service users' views of psychiatric nurses. *Br J Nursing* 1991, 3:16–17.

Roland M, Coulter A. Hospital referrals. *Oxford Gen Pract Series* 1992, 22:6–10.

Rowan KM, Kerr JH, Major E, McPherson K, Short A, Vessey MP. Intensive Care Society's APACHE II study in Britain and Ireland. I: Variations in case mix of adult admissions to general intensive care units and impact on outcome. *Br Med J* 1993, 307:972–81.

Sainio S, Jarvenpaa A-L, Kekomaki R. Thrombocytopenia in term infants: a population-based study. *Obstet Gynecol* 2000, 95:441–4.

Schrader H, Stovner LJ, Helde G, Sand T, Bovin G. Prophylactic treatment of migraine with angiotensin converting enzyme inhibitor (lisinopril): randomised, placebo-controlled, cross-over study. *Br Med J* 2001, 322:19–22.

Shinton R, Sagar G. Lifelong exercise and stroke. *Br Med J* 1993, 307:231–4.

Staessen JA, Byttebier G, Buntinx F, Celis H, O'Brien ET, Fagard R. Antihypertensive treatment based on conventional or ambulatory blood pressure measurement. *J Am Med Assoc* 1997, 278:1065–72.

Treasure J, Schmidt U, Troop N *et al*. First step in managing bulimia nervosa: controlled trial of therapeutic manual. *Br Med J* 1994, 308:686–9.

Turnbull D, Holmes A, Shields N *et al*. Randomised, controlled trial of efficacy of midwife-managed care. *Lancet* 1996, 348:213–19.

Wannamethee SG, Lever AF, Shaper AG, Whincup PH. Serum potassium, cigarette smoking, and mortality in middle-aged men. *Am J Epidemiol* 1997, 145:598–607.

Yong L-C, Brown CC, Schatzkin A *et al*. Intake of vitamins E, C, and A and risk of lung cancer. *Am J Epidemiol* 1997, 146:231–43.

Zoltie N, de Dombal FT, on behalf of the Yorkshire Trauma Audit Group. The hit and miss of ISS and TRISS. *Br Med J* 1993, 307:906–9.

INDEX

The tables and figures listed below have been reproduced from the references indicated.